GROWING TOGETHER

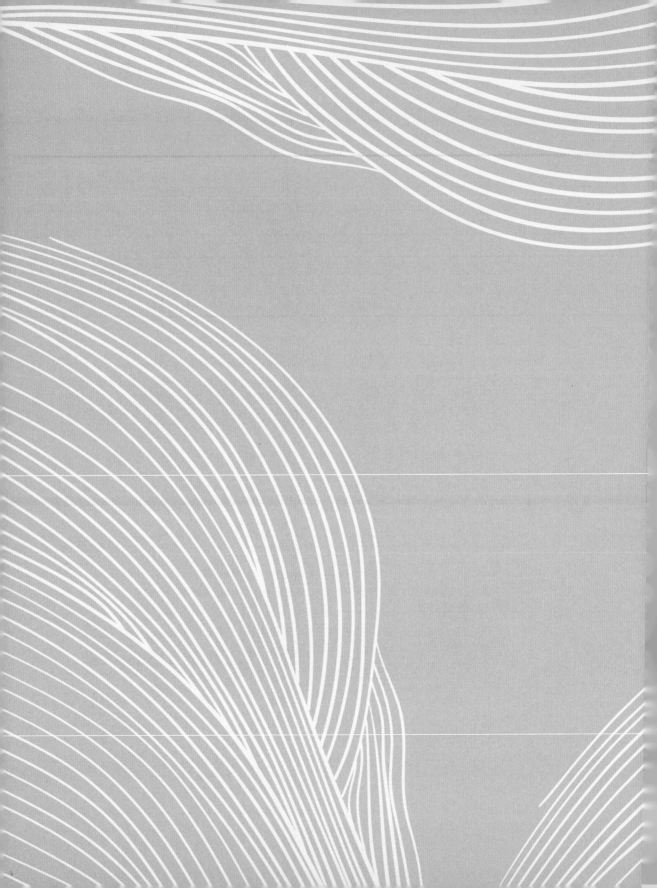

DOULA WISDOM &
HOLISTIC PRACTICES
for PREGNANCY,
BIRTH & EARLY
MOTHERHOOD

A WEEK-BY-WEEK
COMPANION

GROWING TOGETHER

Carson Meyer

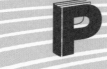

CHRONICLE PRISM

This book contains advice and information relating to health and interpersonal well-being. It is not intended to replace medical or psychotherapeutic advice and should be used to supplement rather than replace any needed care by your doctor or mental health professional. While all efforts have been made to ensure the accuracy of the information contained in this book as of the date of publication, the publisher and the author are not responsible for any adverse effects or consequences that may occur as a result of applying the methods suggested in this book.

Library of Congress Cataloging-in-Publication Data available.

ISBN 978-1-7972-3073-3

Manufactured in China.

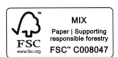

Illustrations by Ellen Heck.
Design by Lizzie Vaughan.
Typesetting by Wynne Au-Yeung.
Typeset in Cormorant Garamond and Gilroy.

10 9 8 7 6 5 4 3 2 1

Chronicle books and gifts are available at special quantity discounts to corporations, professional associations, literacy programs, and other organizations. For details and discount information, please contact our premiums department at corporatesales@chroniclebooks.com or at 1-800-759-0190.

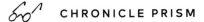 CHRONICLE PRISM

Chronicle Prism is an imprint of Chronicle Books LLC,
680 Second Street, San Francisco, California 94107
www.chronicleprism.com

TO JOHNATHAN & LOU,
THANK YOU FOR MAKING EVERY
DAY A DREAM COME TRUE.

19

FIRST TRIMESTER

87

SECOND TRIMESTER

153
THIRD TRIMESTER

253
FOURTH TRIMESTER

THE FIRST 100 DAYS

INTRODUCTION

I didn't always know about my body's innate ability to create life in health and harmony. As a little girl, I traced my finger over my mother's Cesarean scar, knowing that my body came from hers and that there were sacrifices she made to give me life. In middle school sex ed, the focus was on how not to get pregnant, there were the fragmented pieces I had been told about my own entry into the world, and Hollywood's depictions of a screaming woman with her legs flailing in the air while a masked man covered in blood "delivered" her baby to her. Rather than feeling connected with my birthright as a woman, so much of what informed my relationship with birth was fear: fear of the unknown, fear of surrender, fear of losing life as I knew it.

In a child development class at NYU, I was assigned to watch *The Business of Being Born*, a documentary about giving birth in America. It was the first time I'd ever seen live footage of an "unscripted" birth. This film gave me an entirely new understanding of the strength of women and the sacredness of birth, and it opened my eyes to the grim realities of our health care system. The United States maternal health system is cravenly beholden to insurance companies' bottom lines. Profit and fear of liability often comes before what is in the best interest of mothers and babies. Only in the past century have we turned away from the midwifery model that places women at the center and turned the inherent strength of childbirth into an "illness" that disconnects women from their bodies.

Cesarean rates in the United States[1] are up from 6 percent in the 1970s to 32 percent in 2023. The United States has the highest maternal mortality rate among developed countries,[2] which is particularly high for Black women due to widespread racial bias. The United States government spends $1.2 billion[3] annually on maternity care, and American families pay more to give birth than any other nation.[4] These financial investments are not resulting in improved birth outcomes or satisfaction. The CDC states that one in five women report mistreatment during maternity care.[5] Birth itself is not becoming increasingly dangerous—it is unnecessary intervention leading to high Cesarean rates[6] that creates risk of complications, lack of support, and the disregard for physiological birth that has pushed us in this direction. Physiological birth describes a birth led by the innate human capacity of the woman and her baby, undisturbed by interventions.

The discovery of what birth could be and how profoundly important a healthy motherhood journey is to our civilization inspired me to become a birth doula at twenty-two years old, propelling me to become my own greatest advocate and build my life around inspiring others to do the same. Over the past decade, I've had the privilege of supporting hundreds of parents through pregnancy and birth and becoming a mother myself. My experiences as a doula and parent have helped liberate me from what I once feared about this journey and allowed me to approach my own matrescence with ease.

Michel Odent, a revered French obstetrician, once said, "To change the world, we must first change the way the babies are being born." The way we are born and the way we give birth have a powerful impact on us and our world at large. Pregnancy and birth may be short compared to the lifetime of parenthood that comes afterward, but this sacred time lays the foundation for how we approach motherhood on the other side. A supported mother who is respected in her autonomy is not only less likely to experience birth trauma or postpartum depression but will also feel better equipped to show up with all that she has to give. Being trusted to birth on your own terms can be a catalyst for healing from societal constraints. The imprinting that takes place for a child in the womb on the day they are born and the days and weeks that follow informs their worldview and lifelong physical and mental health far more than we may realize.

The womb is our very first ecosystem. Like Mother Earth, it is perfectly designed to nourish us and provide us with everything we need to thrive. When we tend to ourselves and to our environment with respect, the healthier we all become. After years working as a doula, I was shocked to learn how rare it was for doctors to talk to clients about good nutrition, healthy lifestyle practices, and environmental health. Unfortunately, preventive health through nutrition and lifestyle are seldom taught in medical school.[7] Most prenatal visits with an OB are under fifteen minutes, and postpartum care is nonexistent in the obstetric model. The impacts of a healthy lifestyle for mom and baby are well studied and should be a central point of prenatal and postpartum care.

This week-by-week companion is for you to turn to from conception through the first one hundred days after birth as a holistic resource. Giving birth is not a medical event; it is a sacred one. There is no moment more divine, no time we are more connected to nature and to our spiritual selves. With so much focus on analyzing, we often forget to honor the unknown and to connect with the remarkable life inside. There is an important place for evidence in this conversation, and I draw from research often in my work and throughout this book.

However, one of the greatest lessons we face as we cross the threshold into parenthood is the fact that we don't always have the answers to the many questions that come up along the way, and that's okay.

There are convincing arguments and evidence to back up any point of view, but the approach I am most interested in is the one that is authentically aligned with your heart, your inner wisdom, and your connection with your baby. We don't need to rely on data or medical advice to parent. Birthing and raising children has long preceded modern research. When we operate against our intuition because an expert told us XYZ, we are not mothering from our highest potential.

We often define the start of motherhood as the day our child is born, but I believe that mothering begins before birth and that there is so much we can do during pregnancy to connect with our maternal instincts. Since my daughter Lou was conceived I've felt her sweet presence. Our beginning has been harmonious and I believe this has much to do with the preparation, perspective, and support my work as a doula has afforded me and the focus I put toward a healthy pregnancy, birth, and the postpartum period. Conscious pregnancy practices are an investment for the future of a child and the world at large.

These pages are inspired by the parents I have worked with and my personal motherhood journey. This book can be read week by week or at whatever pace you choose. Each week contains food for thought, stories, resources from professionals I admire, and activities to prepare your mind and body for birth and beyond. Whether this is your first pregnancy or you've given birth before, this book is here to help you feel rooted in your inner voice and wisdom.

MY BIRTH STORY

I have always viewed the women I serve as my teachers. With each birth I witnessed, and each story I heard, I humbly realized how mysterious birth is. Although giving birth is possibly the most universal experience there is, I have found that each and every person's journey holds something unique. Hearing different perspectives helped me challenge the current cultural narratives around birth and my own assumptions. I hope that reading mine does the same for you.

One of the first things I tell my clients is, "Forget your due date. Babies come on their own time, and putting a date to it is only going to get in your head, creating unnecessary expectation or even unnecessary intervention. Surrender to the mystery!" Well, my due date happened to be my twenty-ninth birthday and of course I didn't take my own advice. I was so excited by this sweet coincidence that I looked forward to my birthday in an entirely new way. I was born two weeks "late" and I know that the attachment to an estimated date ultimately contributed to the way that I was born. My mother was induced when she was forty-two weeks pregnant with me. Letting go of the expectation around time was part of processing my own entry into this world in preparation for giving birth.

Although I loved being pregnant and felt physically very comfortable, patience was not easy for me. When my due date came and went, I, like so many before me, wondered if I'd ever go into labor. Like standing on the edge of a cliff, I so badly wanted to jump because I knew that there was no turning back, and diving in seemed far easier than sitting with all the big feelings of anticipation.

I chose to give birth in an environment that would not impose a deadline or expiration date on my pregnancy with a midwife who would support us on our own time. Letting Lou choose her arrival time was important to me, especially knowing that the hormones of labor are initiated by the baby.[8]

A few days after my "due date," I made an effort to stop moping around the house impatiently. My girlfriends made me a killer playlist to lift my spirits and dance on the treadmill. I walked at least a mile every day in the third trimester, but on this day I put some pep in my step. I took photos of my belly, not knowing this would be the last photo before my water broke. My husband, Johnathan, and I were sitting on the couch cuddling with our Bernedoodle, Paulie, about to watch *The White Lotus* when I felt a pop followed by a gush.

My waters released at 8:00 p.m. on the dot. I jumped up in shock and excitement, my heart pounding. We were now on our way to greeting our baby, although I knew we could still be days away! For some, labor begins right after water breaks; for others, it doesn't start for hours or days. In some rare cases it never breaks at all! Ruptured membranes before labor starts is often a path to induction when birthing in the hospital, but being induced immediately is not necessary in most cases and can lead to cascading interventions and risks.

I asked Johnathan to make lentil soup so we would have something nourishing and warm prepared for labor and after birth. I told him to try to get some sleep while he could. We got into bed early knowing it could be our last chance to sleep for some time. Around midnight, I started to feel those first rhythmic waves. They weren't painful but they were consistent and required movement. I rested on my side and swayed against the edge of the bed. By sunrise things were picking up, and although I felt it was too early for my midwife to come, I was craving female energy. Johnathan was tired and I could tell he could use the extra support. We called her around 6:30 a.m. and she arrived an hour later.

As the sun came up over the Blue Ridge Mountains, I remember taking a photo in between waves because I wanted to remember the sunrise on the day our baby would be born. We listened to music, had some soup, and swayed around. In the space between contractions, we chatted, and when a wave took over, my midwife or Johnathan would apply pressure to my hips. My dog, Paulie, stayed glued to my side, looking helpless and concerned. I wore the strand of beads around my neck from my birth blessing ceremony infused with the blessings and love from my friends and family. Even though we chose not to tell anyone I was in labor, I felt them with me every step of the way.

A couple of hours later I got into the shower. Intensity was building, but I was still coping okay. I have very little recollection of what happened in this phase. Much like a fever dream, I would flow in and out of consciousness, or as my dear friend and mentor says, "I left my body to get my baby."

There was no talk of time, no timing of contractions, no cervical exams. Just patience. Just trust. Our midwife and Johnathan steadily and quietly witnessed my process unfolding just as it needed to. Around noon, I insisted on getting into the tub, and from there things really shifted. I no longer felt contractions; instead, I felt the expanding of my hips and tension shooting through the front of my legs. I could feel Lou's head pushing against my tailbone. I wanted someone to just break my tailbone off to put a stop to it. I howled with each contraction. There was no hypnobirthing, no orgasmic birth—just roaring and profanities contrasted against the Vedic chants playing in the background. The perfect encapsulation of birth if you ask me: a beautiful spiritual journey and a real bitch.

Johnathan stayed at my side, steady as a rock. (Even when I bit through his skin.) What grounded me the most and got me through was my connection with Lou. After screaming in agony I would talk to her and tell her that it was all okay and how proud I was of her. I knew she was working hard with me and for that, I was grateful. We were all alone and in it together at the same time.

So much doubt came up in me. I forgot everything I believed about birth. Although I could feel with my fingers that Lou was close, I was convinced it just wouldn't work. When I was sixteen years old at my first gynecologist visit, I was told by the doctor that my petite stature would make it very challenging for me to give birth vaginally one day. I would probably need a Cesarean, she said. Years later, the doula in me knew how bogus this assertion was and that she had no way of accurately predicting that ten years prior to pregnancy, or during pregnancy for that matter. Yet, her voice rang in my ear through each contraction. Perhaps she was right, I thought. Perhaps my body was not fit for birth. I was determined not to let this seed of doubt germinate and overpower all that I knew to be true in my heart. I was at my edge. In retrospect, I was pushing but I had no idea. My body had taken over.

After a couple of hours in the tub, the water was no longer serving me and I wanted OUT. I crawled into bed and draped myself over Johnathan's shoulders. For the next hour my body moved instinctively to make way for Lou. I got onto all fours with my right leg bent up by my right hand. Johnathan placed his hands below her emerging head ready to catch. Once her head was out, she took her first breath and cleared her lungs with a cry. Nobody pulled her out but instead patiently allowed the next contraction to rotate her shoulders and free her body. With the next wave she emerged into her father's hands and was passed under my legs up to me. She was born at 3:50 p.m. Although we waited to find out, I had a strong feeling she was a girl my entire pregnancy (I even filled her closet with my childhood dresses). "It's her!" we said, laughing. I knew all along! Paulie, who had been under the bed, popped up in celebration, doing laps around the room.

Just like our labor, the moments following her birth were completely undisturbed. We let the physiological process unfold as we had through pregnancy and labor. The bliss I had been waiting for arrived and we were soaring with oxytocin. Nobody "stimulated" her, suctioned her, or touched her at all besides the two of us. Nobody "massaged" my uterus to prevent bleeding, cut her cord, or tugged at the placenta. These were things I've seen done unnecessarily and without consent far too often and it broke my heart every time.

After an hour of cuddling, Johnathan cut the cord. I still had to birth the placenta and I was nervous. This was the final stage of birth that needed to happen safely. My midwife intuited that I was on edge about it and resisting any support in guiding it out. She asked if I wanted to squat in the shower to birth my placenta alone. She placed a bowl between my legs and I spoke to the placenta, thanking it for taking such good care of Lou, for being the source of her nourishment and protection. I told my placenta that its work was done and I guided it out with ease. Our midwife put fresh sheets on the bed, warmed up some freshly made lentil soup, and Lou and I fell asleep in each other's arms just as the sun set over the Blue Ridge Mountains.

Looking back, it's true what they say—you forget the pain and it all becomes a blur. I am reminded of what I was taught on my first day of doula training: "A mother may not remember the details of her birth, but she will always remember the way she was treated." With each day that passes my memory fades a little bit more, but I know that the love and reverence Lou and I were shown will forever impact our lives. My hope is that every woman emerges from the most epic transformation of her life feeling stronger than ever before and held by the love and support of her village. May this book be a tool for you in setting yourself up for success in pregnancy, birth, and beyond.

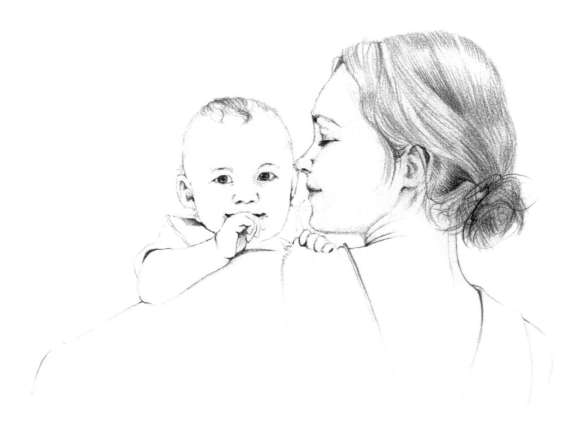

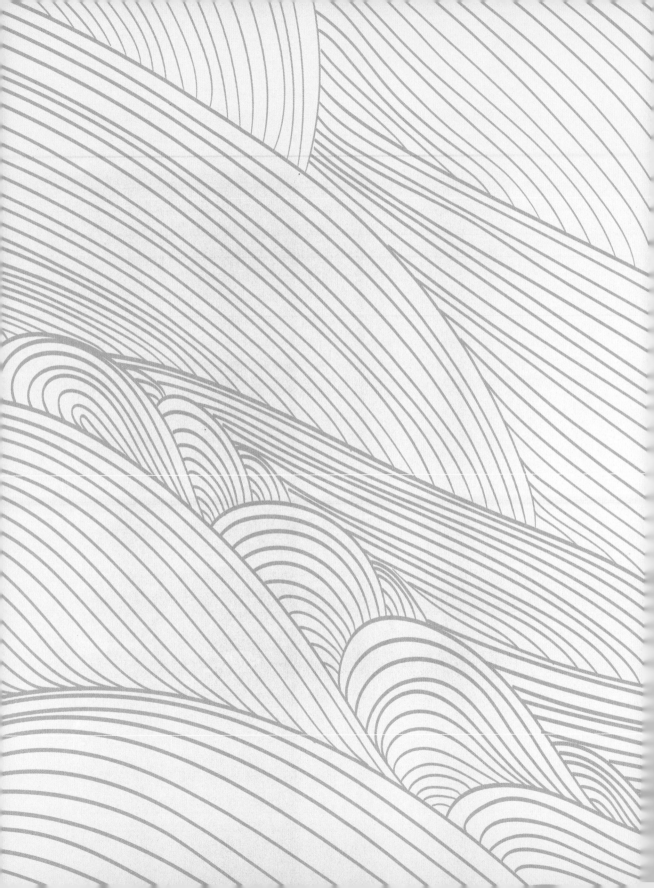

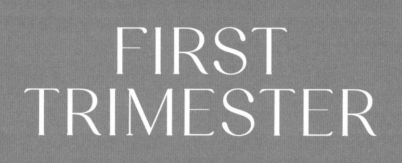

FIRST TRIMESTER

"And as life began in the sea, so each
of us begins his identical life in a miniature
ocean within his mother's womb."

RACHEL CARSON —— *THE SEA AROUND US*

Week 4

THE SACRED BEGINNING

If you are reading this and just found out you're pregnant, congratulations and welcome to a time of transformation and expansion that will change you forever. If you feel nervous about celebrating or jumping for joy this early on, you're not alone. It is hard to put into words the feeling that arises within the early days of pregnancy. I will never forget the butterflies I felt looking down at that first positive pregnancy test. The rush of adrenaline poured through my body, my heart pounding out of my chest followed by a wave of disbelief, joy, doubt, fear, relief, and then one thousand questions storming into my head all at once.

Pregnancy length is calculated from the first day of your last period. Although you likely conceived two weeks ago, you are now considered to be four weeks pregnant! No one told me how long the two weeks between ovulation and the missed period would feel when trying to get pregnant. Wouldn't it be nice if we could test for pregnancy moments after sex? As much as my eager heart and mind would have loved to get an answer right away, I knew that there was a potent lesson for me in sitting with the unknown.

We know how babies are made and yet there is still so much mystery in the process. Some women get pregnant their very first try; others try for years and endure so much heartbreak along the way. Of course, there are physical factors involved in the ability to conceive and carry a pregnancy, but there are also emotional components we tend to overlook. I have worked with countless couples who have tried to get pregnant for years feeling completely hopeless, some who have even sought out fertility treatments to no avail, and then after a major emotional life shift, it happens naturally! These stories are all around us and an important reminder that the spiritual act of growing, birthing, and raising a child cannot simply be reduced to a biological event.

I believe babies choose their parents and that they also choose their timing. One of the biggest lessons we face as parents is the realization that the life you are bringing in is not here to fit into your timeline. Each child is on their own unique life path, just as you are on yours. When a child is conceived, when a baby chooses to be born, when a baby learns to crawl, walk, talk, when they sleep through the night— we have very little control over any of it. We as parents are here simply to hold our children with love and guidance along the way. For many, the patience required in becoming pregnant is the very first initiation into motherhood, preparing us to let go of the expectations we have placed on ourselves and our unborn child.

Parenthood changes our relationship to time in almost every way and expands our capacity for patience more than we may have previously thought possible. These first weeks contain so much expansion in every sense of the word. Your heart is literally working harder, and your blood volume is already increasing.[9] Some early pregnancy sensations may arise, like shortness of breath, increased blood flow and heart rate, nausea, bloating, food aversion, constipation, breast tenderness, and increase in appetite. You might even be having vivid dreams. If so, I invite you to write them down as soon as you wake. Some women don't feel much at all in the early weeks and that is also totally normal! Try not to read into anything too much. There is no one right way to feel emotionally or physically.

You might be wondering, What now? Who do I tell? Will it last? You, like so many mamas before you, may have experienced a previous pregnancy loss and know how it feels to grieve this new love and all the excitement that came with it. It is so common for women to feel concern about how their pregnancy is unfolding and if this baby is here to stay. Take all the time you need before sharing the news, but I invite you to let the pregnancy sink in and to embrace joy in this present moment. There are no guarantees in life and we may be confronted with grief at any given moment, pregnant or not. Parenthood is often described as wearing your heart outside of your body. The vulnerability of loving someone so deeply can feel terrifying. Try not to let the fear keep you from being present and soaking in these sacred early days.

Whether you are a parent already, have been trying to get pregnant for a long time, or this pregnancy came as a surprise, your journey to this moment undoubtedly has an impact on what you are feeling today. You are sandwiched between your lived experience and your anticipation for all that the future holds. I invite you to tune into the moment you are in right now. Let all that has come before and all that will come after fall away while you ground yourself in the present moment. Take a deep belly breath. Notice where the jitters exist in your body. Notice where you are holding tension and where your mind wants to wander. To ground you in the current moment, it may help to identify objects around you. What color are your shoes? What texture is the floor? When we do this, we guide our minds into focusing on what is tangibly in front of us and the safety of the moment we are in. Drop in and allow yourself to truly feel this profound moment.

NOTE

We waited to find out whether we were having a boy or a girl. It was a very special surprise! Throughout the book I will be switching back and forth between "he" and "she" when referring to your baby so just go ahead and change the pronoun to the one that pertains to your baby if you didn't wait to find out.

SHARING THE NEWS WITH FRIENDS AND FAMILY

For some it can feel special to keep this news to yourselves and to be in the intimacy of your big-little secret before the external excitement rushes in. There will come a time when everyone knows, but for now it's yours to keep close if you want to.

With that said, the notion that we must keep pregnancy a secret in the first trimester is largely based around superstition, fear, and the cultural shame and discomfort we have with grief. For many, sharing the news early is important to get the kind of support you may need, and if sharing early resonates with you, don't let old paradigms dictate your path. You deserve the love and support of those around you regardless of the viability of the pregnancy.

Calling in Your Spirit Baby

Years before we made the conscious choice to conceive, I felt the call to motherhood. I'm sure this feeling started to emerge in me because of a combination of factors. I was in my mid-twenties and my biological clock was nudging me, I was in love with a man I knew I wanted to start a family with, and I could feel my daughter's spirit hovering close by. This became especially apparent to me after reading *Spirit Babies*, a book that brings comfort to parents on their fertility journey.

When this feeling emerged, we acknowledged it, but we also wanted to plant roots in the place we were going to live before acting on it. I used that time to write letters to this soul I felt knocking at the door. When we found our home in North Carolina and we were ready to invite a baby to join our family, I wrote this spirit a letter to let her know that we were ready and that she had so much to look forward to here on Earth as a part of our family. I was not surprised when we got pregnant right away. She had been patiently waiting for us to be ready.

I have my clients do this activity whether they are currently pregnant or trying to conceive. It can be done at any and every stage along the way.

WRITE A LETTER TO YOUR BABY

Tell your baby why you are excited to be her mother. What do you want your baby to know about the family she is coming into? What are some of the greatest parts of being here on Earth? How are you preparing for her arrival? What does she have to look forward to in the family she is joining?

NUTRIENTS TO CONSIDER IN THE FIRST TRIMESTER

I became a nutrition consultant a few years into my career as a doula because I knew it would be one of the greatest tools I could offer my clients to support them through pregnancy and the postpartum period. Not only can most pregnancy symptoms (nausea, swelling, and heartburn, to name a few) be alleviated through diet and supplementation, but good nutrition can also decrease the likelihood of and help manage conditions such as gestational diabetes,[10] anemia,[11] and preeclampsia.[12] Optimal maternal diet during pregnancy and breastfeeding have lifelong benefits for mother and child.[13]

CHOOSING A PRENATAL VITAMIN

With thousands of prenatal multivitamin brands and formulas on the market, it can be difficult to know how to decipher which prenatal vitamin will offer the greatest benefits. There are endless amounts of supplements marketed toward pregnant women that not only contain insufficient dosage but also contain ingredients with known contraindications for pregnancy. Since it is impossible to compact the necessary nutrients into a single pill, it is best to choose a prenatal vitamin with a multi-capsule dosage instead of a one-a-day. The next thing I look at is the "additional ingredients" section. Is the product packed with sugar, food coloring, or hydrogenated oils? Steer clear of ingredients like aspartame, silicon dioxide, and monosodium glutamate (MSG), to name a few.

My top prenatal recommendations contain choline, an important nutrient for brain development, and methyl-folate or folate (instead of folic acid), and are formulated without iron. Iron is a heavy metal and although adequate iron levels are important for a healthy pregnancy, too much can be problematic, which is why I recommend it is supplemented on an individual basis and with food first.

You may be wondering why such a strong emphasis is placed on prenatal multivitamins when generations of women before us got by without them. Are they really necessary? There are differing perspectives on this, and some would argue that a densely nutritious diet can and should suffice. I don't completely disagree. What is worth taking into consideration is that a majority of people are eating the "standard American diet" of processed foods, inflammatory oils, and chemical additives, which lead them to nutrient deficiencies that impact pregnancy and postpartum health. Conventional farming practices, widespread use of pharmaceuticals, and deteriorating soil have reduced nutrient levels in our food and impacted our ability to absorb nutrients optimally. In short, in the world we live in today, most mothers could benefit from quality supplementation (prenatal multivitamin or individual supplements) in conjunction with good nutrition.

Below is a list of just a few of the many vitamins and minerals that play a key role in the first trimester. It is crucial to remember that prenatal vitamins do not take the place of a healthy diet. Good nutrition is the best way to support your growing baby and body.

Folate: Folate is an important nutrient for the first trimester for reducing risk of miscarriage, preeclampsia, neural tube defects, and lip and tongue ties. However, folic acid, the synthetic form of folate often used in supplements, does not cross the placenta the way methylated folate does and must be converted by the body to be utilized properly. This is why I do not recommend supplementing with folic acid. Sixty percent of women have the MTHFR gene mutation[14] that interferes with the absorption process, making it especially beneficial to look for folate, methylated folate, or folinic acid when choosing a prenatal vitamin.[15] • Where to find it: *Beef liver, lentils, beans*

Choline: Choline is essential for baby's brain development, and some studies show it may even play a role in enhancing memory function.[16] Choline also supports maternal liver function and placenta health. According to the National Health and Nutrition Examination Survey,[17] 90 percent of women are not meeting their need for choline.[18] Meanwhile, choline is left out of most prenatal multivitamins on the market.

• Where to find it: *Pasture-raised egg yolks, liver, salmon*

Vitamin A: Vitamin A is crucial to the development of fetal facial features, and it also supports the maternal immune system, metabolism, thyroid function, and skin health.[19] Beta-carotene is the form of vitamin A found in plant food sources. It must be converted to preformed vitamin A in the body; therefore, it is less bioavailable than active vitamin A from animal sources. • Where to find it: *Liver and grass-fed butter (active, preformed vitamin A), sweet potato, carrots, and pumpkin (beta-carotene)*

Zinc: Zinc is a mineral that helps support immune function, reduce risk of miscarriage and low birth weight, and may even reduce risk of chronic disease for future generations. Around 80 percent of pregnant women worldwide have inadequate levels of zinc. To maximize absorption of zinc in plant foods, soak, sprout, and/or ferment them. • Where to find it: *Oats, beef, pumpkin seeds*

DITCH THE DUE DATE

Regardless of whether you are certain of your conception date or not, it will serve you to detach from the idea that there is a set day or even week that your baby will arrive. The mystery of a baby's arrival time is another way in which Mother Nature invites us to let go of our attachment to expectation and control. Five percent of babies are born on their due date. In one study, 81 percent of people having their first baby went past their due date and 61 percent of second, third, or later pregnancies went beyond their due date.[20] That's why I prefer to talk about the anticipated arrival time as a "due range" or "birth season." When people ask your due date, practice giving a time range instead of a single date. This not only helps you detach from the guess date but also helps friends and family do the same. Trust me, when that arbitrary date comes and goes you will be bombarded with other people's anticipation, which can be agitating when layered on top of your own eagerness.

29

We all know that babies don't have a calendar or clock in the womb, but the obstetrical model tends to take these estimated due dates quite literally when advising patience. Induction is at an all-time high and many doctors in the United States actually recommend evicting babies a week before the forty-week mark.[21] This is problematic not only because it is based on faulty evidence (more about this in Week 30) but also because cycle length varies from woman to woman and many are not certain of their conception dates altogether.

Choosing the support you have through pregnancy and the postpartum period is perhaps one of the most important factors in setting yourself up for a positive birth experience. If honoring your baby's timeline is important to you, you will want to be sure you are working with a provider who shares that approach.

With each week I will be providing you with prompts and information that will help you reflect on what kind of support is important to you. At no point should you feel trapped with a care provider who isn't the right fit. Although it may take some extra effort, it's never too late to make a switch. I invite you to keep an open mind and explore what all options look like. Before we dive into the pros and cons of the different models of care available to you, I want to share with you about what a birth doula is and how you can utilize the support of a birth doula for an optimal pregnancy, birth, and the postpartum experience.

WHAT IS A BIRTH DOULA?

The word *doula* is a Greek term meaning "servant to a woman," but today it is used to describe someone whose work is to be of service to a woman through pregnancy, birth, and the initial postpartum period.

As a doula I offer resources and education to my clients in pregnancy. I am also available for emotional and physical support throughout. This may look like offering tips on alleviating discomforts that arise in pregnancy and the postpartum period or helping to navigate the many choices parents have to make. I join my clients who are in labor at their home or at the hospital. I have worked with women through all types of births, from planned Cesareans and medicated and unmedicated hospital births to home births and everything in between. The role may look different depending on the clients' needs, but it is always rooted in honoring the individual needs of the mother.

Doulas are often considered advocates for their clients. I struggle with this description of doula support because I believe my clients are all capable of being their own best advocate and by doing so they step into a crucial superpower needed for motherhood. I am there to offer the resources, information, reassurance, and encouragement so that they feel empowered to use their own voice. I will always stand alongside them, to echo their needs and ensure they are being heard. No mother should have to defend herself during the most physically and spiritually intense moment of her life. This is why I am so passionate about preparing families for birth, so that they can be armed with information to build a supportive birth team and be able to confidently navigate whatever comes their way.

Although the benefits of doula support are evidence based, only about 6 percent of women in the United States use one in labor. A 2017 study found that when mothers have the support of a doula, they are more likely to have better birth outcomes.[22] This includes more positive feelings about childbirth, more likely to have a spontaneous vaginal birth, less likely to utilize medication, and a reduced risk of postpartum depression. In addition, their babies are less likely to have low Apgar scores at birth.

How do I find a doula?

Most people find a doula via word of mouth. Friends, local yoga studios, acupuncturists, and birth accounts you follow on social media will likely be able to point you in the right direction.

Should I look for a certified birth doula?

Asking a doula about her training is a good interview question but certification is not necessary. In recent years, agencies have formed with the intention to create clear-cut definitions of what a doula offers within her scope of practice. These certifying bodies may give a doula a stamp of approval on her résumé or website but can also be problematic, especially because we do not perform any medical or clinical tasks. Unlike a licensed professional, doulas have always and should always exist outside the scope set by anyone but herself and the family she is serving. Doulas do not answer to governing organizations, hospitals, doctors, or midwives. We serve mothers.

When COVID lockdowns began, hospitals across the country closed their doors to doulas and even partners while thousands of mothers were forced to give birth alone. After some hospitals lifted these policies, allowing only certified doulas to be present, it prompted a wider conversation: Why does a doula need to be certified? Women are entitled to birth with the support they choose at home and in the hospital regardless of their training and certifications. A woman should be able to have the support of a hired doula or anyone in her life that she wants to fill that role. The pandemic regulations proved that denying mothers support during birth and the postpartum period had an obvious and well-documented impact on maternal stress levels and maternal satisfaction,[23] resulting in greater pregnancy-related complications.[24]

Will my doctor be comfortable with me having a doula?

If your doctor has any objection to you having a doula, that is a serious red flag. They are showing you that they are not interested in collaborative care and are likely practicing in a way that doesn't put mothers' needs at the center. Your doctor should know that the benefits of doula support are evidence based.

When should I hire a doula?

Some couples hire me before they get pregnant, and others hire me in labor (not often, but it has happened). It is never too early or too late to work with a doula, but the sooner you can establish the relationship and build a connection the better. It is also beneficial to be able to lean on her in the early stages of pregnancy.

Do I need a doula if I have a home birth?

When giving birth at home, pain medication is not an option, so doula support can be tremendously helpful in offering hands-on comfort measures and massage. If a transfer takes place, it is also reassuring to know you will have your doula with you to help you navigate that change. A doula can also be a great source of support for your partner at home so that they have an extra set of hands and someone to turn to.

What does a doula cost? Does insurance cover a doula?

Unfortunately, it can be challenging to get insurance to cover doula support, but it's always worth asking. Doula rates vary widely based on location, experience, and what is included in a package. If you are on a tight budget, you may want to interview newer doulas who are looking to gain more experience. There are also many wonderful organizations that can help low-income families get doula support.

I want to use an epidural. Should I still hire a doula?

I have worked with many women who have chosen to get an epidural and still benefit from utilizing doula support. Remember, much of what we do is help our clients become as informed as possible about their choices, and pain management is just one of the many decisions a mama has to make. With an epidural, the strong sensations of labor may be gone but the hard work is not over. A doula will continue to hold loving space and provide encouragement, information, and assistance through birth, initial breastfeeding, and the postpartum period. Having a doula can also help you navigate hospital choices and prevent the cascade of interventions that often comes along with an epidural. (We will chat more about epidurals in week 31.)

What should I ask a doula in the interview process?

Come up with a list of questions that are important to you about how she works and what you can expect from her services. Here are a few good interview questions:

What is your perspective on birth?
How do you help your clients advocate for themselves?
Do you work with a backup?
When do you join your clients in labor?
Are you most comfortable supporting hospital birth, home birth, medicated birth, unmedicated birth?

The most important thing to consider when hiring a doula is how she makes you feel. This person is going to walk with you during the most profound transformation of your life. Your doula should be someone you trust and want to bear witness to your birth. There is a doula for everyone and it's about finding the one that best suits you.

HOW TO CHOOSE THE CARE PROVIDER
THAT IS RIGHT FOR YOU

Doulas work in all different birth environments and support mothers who are under both obstetric and midwifery care. Every doula knows that one of the most important choices her client can make to set herself up for a positive birth experience is choosing the model of care and provider that is most in line with her values and individual birth choices. You are responsible for vetting this person and doing deep reflection to become clear on what is important to you. Although there are factors such as location and insurance coverage that can make switching providers a headache, you should never feel trapped under someone's care. If red flags arise, don't hesitate to make a switch no matter how far along you are in your pregnancy.

Here I have outlined the wide range of care available to you along with some pros and cons to consider. The only right choice is the one that authentically resonates with your needs. To some, freebirth may feel like a radical or unsafe option. To others, non-emergent surgical birth may be seen as extreme or dangerous. Both ends of the spectrum contain benefits and risks. What matters most is that all mothers have a choice and access to the support they desire.

OB-GYN

Location: *Hospital*

An OB-GYN is a trained surgeon specializing in female reproductive health who can perform a wide range of procedures, can prescribe medications, and is skilled in managing high-risk situations.

PROS

+ Usually take insurance (however, you may still leave the hospital with a substantial co-pay)

+ Can easily prescribe medicine and order tests and ultrasounds as needed

+ Specialize in truly high-risk pregnancies and procedures

+ for those who need medical intervention that cannot be offered by a midwife

+ Skilled in performing Cesarean when needed for the well-being of mom and baby

+ Can suture tearing of any degree

CONS

✕ Are skilled in managing high-risk births and emergencies but might not be as well versed in supporting physiological birth

✕ Prenatal visits are brief (typically under fifteen minutes) and wait times can be long

✕ Phone calls are usually directed to a nurse or receptionist

✕ Usually show up at the end of labor (pushing phase) and leave shortly after placenta delivery

✕ Are obligated to practice according to hospital policy where they work and follow the rules and regulations of the medical board

✕ May experience burnout if in a high-volume practice

✕ Six-week checkup after birth; no postpartum care

✕ You are statistically more likely to have an unnecessary medical intervention and Cesarean within the obstetrical care model

✕ Recommendations will usually default to allopathic medicine before offering nutrition, lifestyle, or holistic guidance

Nurse Midwife

Location: *Hospital, home, or birth center*

A nurse midwife is a registered nurse with additional training as a midwife who provides care during pregnancy and birth and is licensed by the state.

PROS

+ Completed nursing school and is well versed in managing clinical or emergent situations that may arise

+ In states that don't recognize midwifery, nurse midwives can practice legally with access to emergency medication

+ Can easily order lab tests and refer out for ultrasounds

+ More likely to accept insurance

+ May provide more time during prenatal visits

CONS

× I would argue that going through nursing school can also be a con. Medical school teaches people how to address emergencies and illness. We need these skills for obvious reasons. However, most pregnancies are not inherently dangerous nor are they a medical event.[25]

× Nurse midwives answer to an attending OB and must practice within the bounds of hospital policy. Nurse midwives who practice at home must follow rules and regulations of their state, which may prevent them from authentically tending to their clients' wishes and needs.

× They often work in a group practice, so you may not know who will be attending your birth

Licensed Midwife (CM/CPM/LM)

Location: *Home or birth center*

A licensed midwife is a trained and board-certified midwife who is skilled in supporting women through pregnancy, birth, and the postpartum period. Licensing varies from state to state.

PROS

+ Can handle most emergencies at home

+ May be eligible for insurance coverage

+ Trained and experienced supporting birth outside the hospital

+ Generally offer more postpartum support within the first days and weeks after birth

+ May offer resources on optimal nutrition, herbal care, and holistic recommendations

+ Legally recognized in some states and therefore may work closely with an OB, is able to refer out for tests, ultrasounds, etc., and has access to emergency medication

CONS

× Are responsible to rules and regulations of the state around home birth and their practice, which may not always align with the best interests of their clients

× May transfer your care at any time that you fall outside of the box (e.g., prior Cesarean, twins, your decline of any test or state-mandated intervention, after forty-two weeks)

× Not legally recognized in every state

Traditional/Autonomous Midwife
Location: *Home*

A lay midwife is an uncertified or unlicensed midwife who often has informal education, such as apprenticeship or self-study.

PROS

+ Practices autonomously and does not have to answer to a medical board or governing agency that dictates how she can care for her clients

+ Specializes in physiological birth at home, and may have the tools and skills to handle emergent situations that may arise

+ Generally offers more postpartum support within the first days and weeks after birth

+ May offer resources on optimal nutrition, herbal care, and holistic recommendations

CONS

✕ Usually does not have relationship with doctor on call if a transfer to the hospital takes place

✕ Not covered by insurance

✕ If a midwife administers medication in an emergency, she could be subject to legal consequences in some states

✕ Training, experience, and skill set will vary, and it should not be assumed that she is trained in emergency interventions

Unassisted/Freebirth

Some choose to give birth without the support of a doctor or a midwife. This is known as an unassisted or freebirth. Freebirth differs from a midwife-assisted home birth in that there is no licensed or formally trained birth professional present.

PROS

+ Undisturbed physiological birth and complete privacy

+ Mother can feel assured that no one will intervene in the birth process

+ Mother has full autonomy over her choices without outside intervention

+ No financial cost

CONS

✕ True emergencies require hospital transfer whereas midwives have skills and tools to respond to most emergencies from home

✕ Although freebirth is legal, one may face legal challenges if an emergency arises

✕ Suturing a tear at home is not an option

✕ Emergency medication is not available

✕ Your partner may not have the support they desire to be present in the birth space

✕ Many women choose this path from an informed and empowered place. However, it may also be chosen because supportive care is not accessible. Every woman should have access to support and the quality of care she desires and should not be left unsupported due to fear of being mistreated by the medical system.

Choosing a provider and birth location is often influenced by a person's risk factors. In a truly high-risk pregnancy or situation with conditions such as preeclampsia, placenta previa, preterm birth, or placental abruption, the safest place to birth is in the hospital with close access to an operating room and emergency interventions.

However, the term high-risk gets thrown around a lot these days and many women feel limited in their choices because of this label. Things like "geriatric" pregnancy (a term I despise) or pregnancy over thirty-five, IVF pregnancy, an over- or underweight mother, twin pregnancy, breech birth, or prior Cesarean may carry higher risks but are not conditions that should automatically risk you out of your desired birth preferences. In my opinion, when the high-risk label is used in the absence of a truly high-risk condition, it creates unnecessary stress and fear that then leads to unnecessary interventions that can create greater risks. If you fall into this category, be mindful of the language you use to describe your pregnancy. Our words hold power.

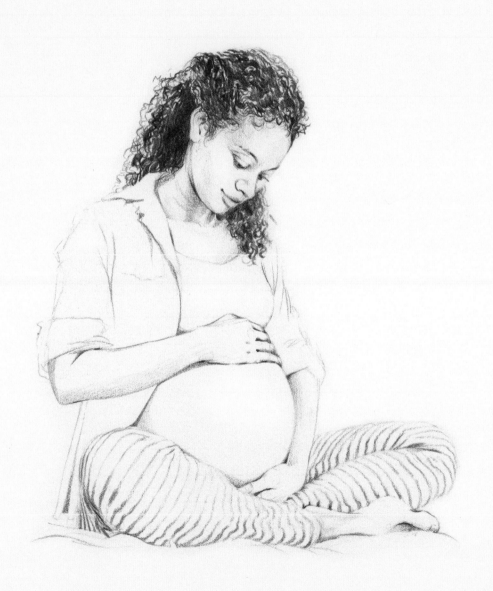

What Does Good Prenatal Care Feel Like?

This week's activity is to journal about what kind of care you want to receive in your pregnancy, birth, and the postpartum period. Focus on how you want to *feel*. The questions below will guide you in reflecting on what is important to you and will help you in the process of finding the right provider for you.

- What does optimal prenatal care look like to you?

- How much time do you get in your visits?

- How easy is it to reach your provider?

- Does your ideal provider offer guidance on dietary and lifestyle health before recommending pharmaceuticals?

- How do they honor your unique needs?

- How does your doctor or midwife respond to your questions and concerns? Do they share horror stories or compare you to other patients in their practice?

- How does your ideal provider approach birth? Do they trust you? Do they recognize your ability to make decisions on your own behalf and for your baby? How do they show you this?

- What kind of language do they use? (Do they say things like "You aren't allowed" or "You can't" or do they practice informed consent?)

- Do they ask your permission before doing a clinical task?

- When you envision yourself giving birth, who is around you?

YOUR INNER LIGHTHOUSE

We are born knowing. Our hearts know how to beat, our bodies know how to move, how to breathe, to cry, to suckle, to sleep. This innate wisdom is not taught to us; it's deeply ingrained within our DNA. Birth and mothering are no different. All we need is already within.

We come into the world with instincts, and we're simultaneously hardwired to gather information from our surroundings for survival. We come to understand life through these lived experiences and shared stories. They help us adapt to the environment we live in and feel a sense of belonging within a community.

For most of us, our perception of birth is informed through what we learn from friends, family, doctors, books, films, and television. Being social creatures, we tend to follow the ways of the tribe, to turn to others for answers. Gathering outside information is an important tool for decision making, but if we aren't using discernment when processing external information, we neglect an equally important

44

source of knowledge that comes from within. We all have an inner lighthouse that helps us navigate. The more we follow this light, the brighter it becomes for us. To tune into this inner light source of knowing we must be open to unlearning, and by that I mean approaching new concepts with a beginner's mind and exploring the sources of our belief systems so we can see our inner light more clearly.

It is helpful to consider these two types of knowing:

Innate Knowing: Our innate wisdom is not something we learned in school or were taught by our parents. It is not governed by our thoughts or influenced by the world around us. It is our nature, hardwired deep within our cells, and works with our inner compass. It cannot always be explained through language and is often felt within the body.

Modern Knowing: Modern knowing is the type of knowing that is found outside of ourselves. It's what we learn from school, stories, doctors, teachers, and research. It is often regarded as superior to innate knowing and considered absolute truth, although it is not. We have become accustomed to believing that we can make sense of the world through modern knowledge and the more we "know" the more we can avoid feelings of uncertainty, danger, or harm.

Taking Inventory

The activity I am going to guide you through will first ask you to take inventory of what you "know" about birth. Take out your journal and freewrite whatever comes to mind when I ask you the following questions.

What are the rights and wrongs you have been taught about birth, the postpartum period, and parenting? What are the images you hold in your mind? What do you know about your own birth into this world? If you've given birth before, how has your previous experience informed your beliefs about birth? How has your mother's birth or the experience of your sister and friends shaped your ideas around childbirth? What cultural natives or expectations influence your perceptions?

Now turn to an empty page in your journal and draw a vertical line through the middle of the page. On the top of the left column write "Innate Knowing" and on the top of the right column write "Modern Knowing." As you read back your reflections, categorize (bullet points will do) what you wrote in the column that best describes the type of knowledge you referenced based on the descriptions below. You may find that one column is more filled out than the other and, in my experience, the modern knowing column is almost always heavier.

This is an activity you can continue to turn to throughout pregnancy to find more balance between the two. Mark this page in your journal and keep expanding on the lists as new information comes to you both internally and externally. As you start to pay more attention to the innate knowing within, this list will reflect that.

EXAMPLE

INNATE KNOWING	MODERN KNOWING
• My body knows how to birth without instruction.	• Ultrasounds can confirm pregnancy and measure the baby.
• My baby knows how to grow inside me.	• I am making this decision based on a study.
• Labor will begin when my baby is ready.	• My doctor said I can't eat or drink in labor.
• My body is telling me to slow down.	• My friends say birth is too painful to bear.

THOSE FIRST TRIMESTER FEELS

By week seven you are likely starting to feel more changes taking place in your body. You may find your sense of smell has heightened or that you're waking up more often to go pee in the night. You may have even noticed that your nipples are already changing in preparation for breastfeeding. Hormones are surging and things are happening. Since last week your baby has doubled in size, arms and legs are sprouting, and your baby's brain is growing 100,000 new cells per minute! In this chapter you can find some of my go-to recommendations for addressing physical changes and challenges that may present themselves in the first trimester.

Nausea in pregnancy impacts 80 percent of women, so if you are in the thick of it you are certainly not alone. For some it's just a queasy feeling and unpleasant taste and for others it is debilitating sickness. We don't have clear-cut answers of why nausea symptoms vary so widely from pregnancy to pregnancy and why 20 percent of women don't experience any nausea at all. However, there are some interesting theories, such as our toxic burden, genetics, hormone imbalance, liver function, stomach bacteria, nutrient deficiencies, and food intolerance. Remember that this is a season and won't last forever. Most start to feel an improvement around twelve weeks of pregnancy.

Although morning sickness is often described as all-day sickness, symptoms tend to be heightened in the morning due to the night-long fast that can impact blood sugar levels. The advice to snack throughout the day is in response to the undeniable correlation we see between low blood sugar levels and nausea. In order to maintain healthy blood sugar levels, you will want to focus on the quantity and quality of the foods you eat as well as exercise and manage stress.

How you start the morning has a big impact on blood sugar levels throughout the day. A well-balanced breakfast should be eaten soon after waking, containing healthy fats and protein-rich foods such as pastured eggs, pastured bacon, grass-fed butter, whole-fat probiotic yogurt, and avocado. Carbohydrates in the form of whole, unprocessed foods such as rice, vegetables, fruit, sweet potatoes, and beans should be consumed with healthy protein and to support stable blood sugar levels. This advice won't just improve nausea but will also have a positive impact on your energy level, sleep, mood, and the long-term health of you and your baby.

It is important not to skip meals or let too much time go in between eating. You may want to consider leaving some nuts, a protein-rich smoothie, or a hard-boiled egg on your bedside table to snack on when you get up to use the bathroom or have a drink of water. This may lead to better sleep and reduced nausea.

Nausea can bring on a vicious cycle where the thought of food makes you feel sick but the absence of it makes you sicker. Do your best and give yourself grace for the season you're in. Your baby is going to get what she needs from the nutrient stores you have. Use any and every opportunity where you feel well enough to eat to nourish yourself with protein-rich foods. Once you are able to get back to equilibrium, replenishing your reserves and nourishing your body through good nutrition will benefit you and your baby through the rest of your pregnancy, the postpartum period, and the breastfeeding journey.

Balanced Meal Ideas

- Pastured eggs (with yolk) soft scrambled with pastured bacon, avocado, and spinach; cooked with grass-fed butter; and topped with sauerkraut

- Breakfast sausage sourced from pastured or grass-fed meats, with a side of watercress (dressed with lemon and olive oil), avocado, and sauerkraut

- Cauliflower rice with homemade pesto and a side of mushrooms sautéed in grass-fed butter with an egg on top

- Spaghetti squash topped with ground liver, beef, and tomato sauce

- Oatmeal soaked in the fridge overnight in coconut milk and chia seeds, then warmed with collagen protein, ghee, cinnamon, chopped almonds, and fresh berries

- Hard-boiled egg with unrefined salt

- White rice with seaweed, wild salmon roe, toasted sesame seeds, and avocado

- Chicken liver pâté on homemade sourdough (Recipe in Week 25)

- Bacon-wrapped dates

- Smoothie with avocado, coconut milk, coconut oil, berries, chia seeds, and collagen protein topped with granola and a dollop of almond butter

Bone Broth

Bone broth is rich in collagen and fantastic for your digestive system, joints, skin, and bones. Try sipping it throughout the day to alleviate nausea. We always keep mason jars of bone broth in the fridge and freezer to use for cooking. It adds great flavor to soups, braises, and beans.

2 lb [910 g] bones from grass-fed/finished or pastured meat

1 onion, halved (with skin)

2 carrots

3 ribs celery

1 Tbsp salt

2 Tbsp apple cider vinegar (this helps draw out the nutrients from the bones)

Add all the ingredients to an Instant Pot and add enough water to fill the PC max line seal. Cook for 120 minutes on high pressure and then natural release for at least an hour. Strain through a fine-mesh sieve into mason jars. Yields about 3½ qt.

51

Store in glass mason jars in fridge or freezer. Leave at least three inches at the top so it can expand safely. The fat cap that forms acts as a seal preventing air to get in, keeping it fresh for longer. Bring to boil before drinking.

Natural Nausea Remedies

Lemon Ginger Juice: Peel and juice a medium-size piece of fresh ginger. If you don't have a juicer you can blend it with water and strain through a fine-mesh strainer. Add the ginger juice to a large mason jar; add water and fresh lemon juice to taste. For electrolytes you can also add a pinch of pink sea salt.

Hydration: In order to stay well hydrated you may want to consider adding electrolytes to your water. Quality is key. Be wary of colored drinks marketed as thirst quenchers that are packed with processed sugar and chemical food dyes. Opt for coconut water or add a pinch of pink sea salt to your water instead. Foods such as watermelon and cucumber that have a high water content are also good for hydration.

Sodium: Contrary to popular belief, seasoning whole foods and balanced meals with unrefined salt is a great way to get minerals into your diet. Optimal sodium levels may improve nausea and are beneficial in helping you stay hydrated. Sodium also improves nutrient absorption, promotes healthy stomach acid, and reduces swelling, headaches, and muscle cramps.

Magnesium: Like salt, magnesium is an essential electrolyte mineral that helps with fetal growth, insulin regulation, digestion, sleep, relaxation, and so much more. Magnesium helps balance blood sugar, which we know can be an important factor in reducing nausea. It also may help relax an overactive gag reflex. You can take magnesium supplements, apply it topically, or enjoy its relaxing effects in a magnesium salt bath.

Vitamin B6: Research has shown that vitamin B6 can help alleviate nausea in pregnancy. Take 25 mg of the active form, pyridoxal-5-phosphate, every eight hours. Be sure to source the active form of B6, pyridoxal-5-phosphate, because some women don't process pyridoxine, which could lead to worsening symptoms.

Hypnosis and Meditation: The use of hypnosis and meditation to manage nausea in pregnancy have been studied[26] and are worth a try. There's no denying that the mind has power over the physical sensations of the body. We also know that meditation can reduce stress and therefore support optimal blood sugar levels.

Homeopathy: Nux Vomica, Sepia Officinalis, and Pulsatilla are homeopathic remedies that are useful for treating nausea.[27]

Movement: Another great way to support blood sugar levels is through gentle exercise or movement. As challenging as it may be to feel motivated to get up and out of the house, it can make a big difference in how you feel. This doesn't have to be anything strenuous; simply a walk around the block, stretching, or gentle yoga is enough to have an impact. Turn to Week 15 for more on exercise during pregnancy.

In working with clients to help manage nausea, I have seen significant improvement with the reduction of industrial seed oils, gluten, processed sugars, refined foods, and even caffeine. Industrial seed oils, or polyunsaturated fatty acids (PUFAs), such as canola, sunflower, vegetable, grape seed, and soybean oil, are found in most processed foods and beverages today and are very different in composition from healthy saturated fats found in grass-fed butter, avocado, fish, and olive oil. Saturated fats deliver healthy skin, hair, and nails; boost brain function and fertility; enrich breast milk; and support a healthy metabolism. Processed and highly oxidized trans fats and seeds oils, on the other hand, create inflammation in the body and are disruptive to hormone production. PUFAs are often hiding in "health foods" such as nut milks and salad dressings and are widely used as cooking oils. When cooking, opt for grass-fed butter, avocado oil, tallow, or ghee instead.

COFFEE IN PREGNANCY

Given the limitations of our understanding of how coffee impacts pregnancy, mothers should pay attention to their individual response to caffeine. Many women will develop aversions in pregnancy or find that avoiding or limiting caffeine intake improves symptoms of nausea. This is likely because caffeine can impact hormones and lead to adrenal stress. We may not know the long-term impact of caffeine on a baby in utero but we do know that it crosses the placenta[28] and can deplete iron and calcium stores. Some studies conclude that even a moderate amount of caffeine can impact the growth of a fetus,[29] which is why I chose to skip it altogether.

CONSTIPATION

Even though your baby isn't taking up much real estate just yet, the shift in hormones like progesterone and relaxin can slow digestion, making constipation common in the first trimester. Prioritize healthy fats in the diet to help lubricate the bowels. Many of the same things that help with nausea will also help with digestion, hydration being an obvious one. Starting your day with warm water and lemon is a great morning ritual that can get things moving. You may also want to consider investing in a squatty potty.

Natural Constipation Remedies

Slippery Elm Bark Powder: This coats the digestive tract and can help stool pass more easily. Although it is contraindicated in pregnancy when inserted into the cervix, it is not known to be adverse when taken orally. Try 1,600 mg of powder mixed in a glass of water before bed. Be sure to take it separately from medications, as it may impact absorption.

Magnesium Citrate: Magnesium is a mineral that plays a vital role in many different physical functions, including metabolic health, cognitive performance, and immune and system regulation. It also works wonders for a myriad of pregnancy-related symptoms, including constipation. Since magnesium can help relax muscles and pull water into the intestines, it can be used to promote healthy bowel movement. There are different forms of supplemental magnesium. Magnesium citrate has the greatest impact on the bowels for alleviating constipation. It can be taken daily to encourage healthy digestion, among other benefits that we will cover later in the book.

REFLUX, INDIGESTION, AND HEARTBURN

Digestive issues can present themselves in many ways as a result of hormone changes and organs shifting to make room for baby. Probiotics, slippery elm, apple cider vinegar (2 to 3 tsp mixed in water) before meals, ginger, and digestive enzymes have been known to alleviate symptoms. You may also want to take inventory of any foods in your diet, such as caffeine, raw veggies, and spicy or acidic foods that may be aggravating to your system.

55

What About Antacids?

Antacids are very frequently recommended to expecting mamas as a safe solution to reflux. However, few women are told the risks and potential side effects of antiacid medication, which should always be taken into consideration before use. Antacids can alter gut bacteria and decrease calcium and vitamin B12 absorption. Since they shift the pH in your stomach, antacids can leave you more susceptible to food-borne illness and infections. They do not address the root cause and may create greater complications. Getting to the source of indigestion through nutritional changes should always be the first step to alleviate reflux before introducing antacids.

FOOD AVERSIONS AND CRAVINGS

I consider cravings to be wisdom from the inner lighthouse leading you to increase necessary nutrients that your baby and body need more of to thrive. That said, external influences can and often do impact how these cravings present themselves. For example, if you're craving ice cream, you won't benefit from high fructose corn syrup, refined sugar, cornstarch or carrageenan found in most store-bought ice creams. However, your body may be telling you it could benefit from more calcium or unrefined healthy fats or is craving sugar to access more energy.

I have worked with many vegans and vegetarians who started craving meat in their pregnancy. This is likely because their bodies are communicating the need for more fat, protein, iron, calcium, folate, zinc, or B vitamins, which is more bioavailable through animal protein. Protein needs rise during pregnancy to build new cells and support the growth of your baby. Amino acids such as taurine, glycine, and carnitine are scarcely found in plant foods, so if you are a vegan or vegetarian and feeling called to introduce animal proteins into your diet, don't ignore that inner wisdom.

I invite you to follow your cravings but always check in with what the craving is communicating and how you can respond to the nutritional need in the healthiest way possible while prioritizing whole foods, made fresh from high-quality sources.

Noelle's Homemade Ice Cream

My friend Noelle Kovary is an Ayurvedic practitioner, herbalist, and bio-energetic nutrition coach turned full-time mama and homesteader. Noelle promotes a slow living and close to nature lifestyle and helps women bust their fears around food to ditch diet culture. Every morning with her babies in tow she milks her Jersey cows to feed her family with fresh raw milk, which contains the bioactive benefits of dairy. Believe it or not, ice cream is a staple food in her healthy family. After all, it is rich in protein, choline, healthy fats, calcium, probiotics, and immuno-globins. Try adding the mixture below to an ice-cream maker.

3 pastured egg yolks

1 cup [240 ml] organic maple syrup

2 cups [480 ml] A2A2 cream

2 cups [480 ml] A2A2 milk

About 20 fresh mint leaves

½ tsp vanilla bean or vanilla extract

Mix egg yolks and maple syrup in a bowl and set aside. Warm cream, milk, and mint leaves in a pot on medium heat (do not let boil) and allow to cool. Add the egg mixture and vanilla to the pot. Warm again briefly on medium-low heat, then let cool completely. You may include chocolate chips to taste.

The Mind-Body Connection

In the 1980s, Dr. Ryke Geerd Hamer established the framework of German New Medicine, which is founded on the belief that all ailments and symptoms correspond to a biological cause and that understanding the emotional stressor is the key to treatment. Although Dr. Hamer's work is considered radical in an allopathic medical model, at its core, it is grounded in the undeniable truth that we are emotional beings. Attempting to isolate the physical body from the emotional self ignores the beautiful complexity of the human experience. I first learned about German New Medicine during my pregnancy after experiencing a recurring rash around my left eye that would appear no matter what changes I made in my diet and skin care routine.

My friend Dr. Maura invited me to tune into what this irritation might be expressing to me and spend some time journaling on my relationship to mothering. How do I view motherhood? How do I experience being mothered? What am I afraid of as I step into this new role? Is there any grief arising with the joy that needs to be felt?

After purge writing my thoughts and feelings, I woke up the next morning and the rash was redder and more irritated than ever before. Dr. Maura reassured me that this was a good indication that energy was moving through. She was right, and by the end of the day it was completely gone and never returned! This was a valuable reminder to me not to resist challenges but view them as a potential to grow.

This week I invite you to explore what motherhood means to you and to give light to any of the feelings that arise within you as you meditate on the identity shift taking place. Take note of any physical symptoms you might be experiencing and how they may be showing up to invite you to deepen your connection with your emotions both past and present.

DISCERNING WITH CONFIDENCE

At two months pregnant, you can't feel your baby fluttering around just yet, but your little one is moving, grooving, and growing a millimeter every day! You may be feeling that first trimester fatigue as your body works around the clock to grow a human. Remember, you are taking part in the ultimate act of creation. Over the past month and change, your body has transformed a mass of cells into a fetus. Regardless of how you're spending your days, the efficiency and hard work you are doing takes an incredible amount of energy. Try not to compare yourself to others or to your pre-pregnancy self. You may be feeling "sluggish," but don't forget that even if you stayed in bed all day, your level of productivity is immeasurable compared to those around you.

Listen to your body and give yourself permission to rest. In a world where we are rewarded for working around the clock and constantly pushing ourselves toward the brink of burnout, rest is something many of us have to consciously practice doing. I often tell my clients that the fatigue that arises in the first trimester is your body asking you to get good at slowing down, to prioritize stillness, and is preparing you for a new pace of life that comes with parenthood.

As a doula, I get a lot of questions about what is safe in pregnancy and what should be avoided. You are probably realizing by now there's so much contradictory advice and pregnancy studies are limited for ethical reasons. A quick Google search will have you running from hot baths, herbal tea, sushi, cheese, coffee, and even your own garden! Pregnant mamas are constantly being told what they "can't" do, but the truth is most of these precautions are not rooted in evidence and can deter women from certain activities that are actually beneficial to their health. It was a profound moment for me in my pregnancy when I asked my midwife if I was "allowed to" take a sauna while pregnant. Her answer was, "I am not in the business of telling women what they can and can't do. You know your body best. You can use your own judgment and discernment to decide."

There's something about being told what we are and aren't supposed to do that is just plain comforting at times. We don't have to over-analyze or feel pressure to make the "right" choice when the decision is made for us. One of the tough, yet liberating, realities about becoming an adult is that we are responsible for ourselves and our choices. No one will ever care more about the well-being of your child than you do. You may not always have all the answers, but when it comes to your body and your baby, there is no expert who knows better than you. It is up to you to take full ownership and responsibility for how you lead your life and raise your children.

Analyzing risks and benefits will never be one-size-fits-all. It is impossible to live life without risks and living in fear strips us of the joy of being in the present moment. However, there is a difference between fear and discernment. Discernment is defined as the ability to judge well, whereas fear is defined as an unpleasant emotion caused by the belief that something is dangerous. Fear does not get you very far, but discernment is a powerful tool to rely on for your mama bear instincts.

Here are some questions (in no particular order) that I use to help me navigate my inner and modern knowing so that I can make informed decisions for my family from a place of confidence:

1   What are the risks or personal concerns to take into consideration? What can I learn from history, traditional use, or other cultures?

2   Are there any benefits?

3   What does my inner wisdom tell me? How does it make me feel?

4   Can I reduce my risk or seek out alternatives?

5   How might fear of judgment be impacting my decision making?

Your Innate & Modern Wisdom, Working Together

These steps don't give you a formula to arrive at an answer; rather, they invite you to think critically and thoughtfully using both your innate and modern wisdom. Practice using these questions as a road map to strengthen your relationship with both sources of wisdom. Notice what a yes feels like in your body and what a no feels like.

EXAMPLE   CONSUMING RAW SUSHI IN PREGNANCY

1 **What are the risks or personal concerns to take into consideration? What can I learn from history, traditional use, or other cultures?**
When considering raw sushi in pregnancy, the primary concern is foodborne illness, parasites, and mercury exposure. Data shows that the risk of foodborne illness from eating sushi and sashimi is higher in countries that don't have legal regulations established regarding the temperature in which the fish is stored. The CDC states that shellfish contributes to 33 percent of parasitic infections but fish only contributes to 0.4 percent and that the fish that are most likely to contain parasites are usually not served raw. For Japanese women, eating sushi during pregnancy is not only customary but recognized as a nutritious part of an expecting mother's diet.

2 Are there benefits?
Fish is a wonderful source of DHA, protein, and fat that helps
support fetal brain development. Fish contains iodine for healthy
thyroid function. It is a nutritious and delicious meal that promotes
stable blood sugar levels. It is also one of my favorite foods and
sparks joy for me!

3 What does my inner wisdom tell me? How does it make me feel?
The benefits and joy of eating sushi in moderation from a high-
quality source outweighed the potential risk. I did not, however, feel
good consuming tuna due to mercury levels or raw shellfish due to
the increased risk of infection. Oysters are one of my favorite foods
and incredibly nutritious, but my concerns took the joy out of the
experience for me during pregnancy.

4 Can I reduce my risk or seek out alternatives?
Steps I can take to reduce my risk include using good judgment
about where I choose to eat sushi, choosing smaller fish to minimize
mercury exposure (lower in mercury), cooking shellfish, always
opting for wild salmon, taking chlorella and selenium to help bind
heavy metals, and avoiding antacids, which alter the stomach pH,
making us more susceptible to foodborne illness.

5 How might fear of judgment impact my decision making?
I definitely got some stares and glares when eating sushi pregnant,
but that didn't concern me because I felt confident in my choice.
It's important that your decision comes from authentic alignment
with what is best for you.

YOU ARE MOTHER EARTH

My mother gave me the name Carson after the ecologist and writer Rachel Carson, whose book *Silent Spring* is credited with advancing the global environmental movement in the 1960s. Rachel Carson's understanding of the detriment caused by pesticide use led to the ban of DDT and the formation of the Environmental Protection Agency. Her work taught us that toxic chemicals magnify as they make their way up the food chain through a process called bioaccumulation and that ultimately it is humans who will suffer the greatest consequences of our environmental recklessness.

I would argue that Rachel Carson's work is one of the greatest contributions to prenatal care, helping us realize that we are all interconnected and only as healthy as the environment around us. She warned that future generations would inherit the consequences of toxic chemical pollution, and she was right. Approximately two hundred man-made chemicals are found in a newborn's cord blood, many of

65

which can be traced back to everyday personal care products, from home cleaning to skin care.

In 2016, the HERMOSA study found that when teenage girls removed endocrine-disrupting chemicals, such as phthalates, parabens, oxybenzone, and triclosan, from their skin care routine, they saw a 25 to 45 percent reduction of these chemicals in their urine after just three days![30] This is just from removing products, without even implementing any detox protocol. This study serves as a great reminder that our choices matter and when not overburdened by pollutants our bodies know how to detox.

I share the following tips because I believe we as individuals can make small changes that improve the health of our families and together create ripple effects of progress. With so much beyond our control, it is more important than ever to limit exposure where we can within our homes and communities.

PLASTICS

Plastic is everywhere we turn, and its durability means it will outlive you and your baby. Not only does plastic pollute our oceans and planet, but it also contains endocrine-disrupting chemicals such as PCPs and BPAs that mimic hormones in the body and can wreak havoc on your reproductive health. Unfortunately, plastic products that are advertised as BPA-free are often replacing BPA with equally harmful chemicals that lack proper safety studies.[31]

Sometimes healthier choices come at a higher price point. As you begin to think about the things you will be purchasing for your baby, consider what you might not actually need. So many lightly used baby items go to the landfill unnecessarily. Think about what items you may want to purchase secondhand or borrow from a friend.

66

Opt for: *Glass baby bottles, glass storage containers, bamboo baby plates, wooden toys, and silicone milk trays for breastmilk storage*

DIAPERS

Speaking of plastic, did you know that most disposable diapers are made with plastic polymers and phthalates? Phthalates are known endocrine disruptors that can alter the functioning of the hormone system, impacting reproductive health and development. Many conventional diaper brands also contain pesticides, formaldehyde, bleach, chlorine, and volatile organic compounds (VOCs), which can cause rashes and skin irritation. Plastic-containing diapers will take five hundred years to decompose in landfills, and about 250 million diapers are thrown away every day.

Opt for: *Reusable diapers, disposable brands that are EWG certified with greener technology and free of chemicals, dyes,[32] and fragrances*

SKIN CARE

Our skin is our largest organ. This organ absorbs what is on and around it and secretes waste as one of our major detox pathways. My own skin sensitivities and healing journey led me to make skin care products in my home kitchen and eventually launch an organic skin care line, C & The Moon. Conscious skin care use is an area of particular importance to me. Once I started working with mothers and babies, I saw firsthand how vital the skin-to-skin connection is for breastfeeding, nervous system synchronization, temperature regulation, and bonding. Babies use touch and smell to familiarize themselves with their mothers and adapt to the world around them. It is imperative that whatever is used on baby's skin is well vetted, and it is equally important that mama is prioritizing clean products too.

67

Opt for: *The Environmental Working Group Skin Deep Database is a great resource for learning more about the safety of specific ingredients in skin care.*

SUNSCREEN

Avoid sunscreens with oxybenzone, avobenzone, octisalate, octocrylene, homosalate, and octinoxate. Oxybenzone is a known endocrine disruptor and most of these ingredients have huge data gaps.

Opt for: *Non-nano particle zinc sunscreen*

FRAGRANCE

Many scented products on the market contain VOCs linked to respiratory health issues and damage to the liver, kidneys, and central nervous system.[33] Plus, fragrances can interfere with your baby's ability to smell you. Babies (and adults) understand the world through their senses and rely heavily on the scent of their mothers to feel safe and to breastfeed. Babies' sensitive systems can become overwhelmed by harsh fragrances, which is why I recommend ditching the regular use of any perfume or strongly scented products (including laundry detergent) through pregnancy, birth, and the first year of your baby's life. You may also want to consider asking caretakers and visitors to do the same.

Opt for: *Unscented products, essential oils, or subtle fragrances formulated with nontoxic ingredients*

HOME CLEANING

Studies show that babies born to mothers who use chemical cleaning products were two times more likely to develop breathing problems.[34]

Opt for: *Get friendly with good old-fashioned vinegar and baking soda. Vinegar is a great alternative for cleaning your windows, bathtub, countertops, and just about anything else in your house. Use baking soda on tile, baths, and counter surfaces. You can add a few drops of essential oils for scent. Teatree oil and lavender both have antimicrobial properties.*

HAND SANITIZERS

Use hand sanitizers and antimicrobial/antibacterial cleaning products sparingly. The overuse of antibacterial ingredients on hands and surfaces contributes to superbugs, bacteria resistant to antimicrobials, and hand sanitizers can increase the absorption rate of some chemicals like BPA. When it comes to washing hands, the use of warm water and soap is sufficient.

LAUNDRY

The number one selling laundry detergent on the market is Tide, which has an F rating on the Environmental Working Groups database. Its ingredients have been linked to skin irritations, allergies, respiratory issues, aquatic toxicity, cancer, and damage to DNA and vision.

Opt for: *Unscented, nontoxic detergent*

KITCHEN

Nonstick cookware is incredibly convenient but comes at a cost. When heated to high temperatures, Teflon releases PFAs and other hazardous toxins into our food and home environment. In 2010, research found higher blood levels of PFOA to be associated with a greater risk of thyroid disease, heart disease, and stroke, even at relatively low levels.

Opt for: *Stainless steel, cast iron, ceramic, and glass*

69

EWG reports that more than 70 percent of non-organic fresh produce sold in the United States contains residues of potentially harmful pesticides.[35] Glyphosate, the key ingredient in Roundup and the most commonly used herbicide in the United States, is toxic to the nervous system, immune system, and gut lining, making humans more susceptible to celiac disease, autism, endocrine disruption, and cancer. Commonly used pesticides have also been linked to attention deficit hyperactivity disorder, or ADHD, in children, whose developing brain and nervous systems are incredibly sensitive to disruption and damage from industrial chemicals.

A 2006 study analyzed the urine of elementary school children who consumed a diet of largely conventional foods. After just five days of an all-organic diet, the levels of malathion and another pesticide, chlorpyrifos, dropped significantly to nondetectable levels. Like the HERMOSA study, this demonstrates the power of positive change when healthier choices are made.

Opt for: *Locally grown, organic food*

MATTRESS

Babies spend half of their first year asleep and adults spend one-third of life sleeping. When we sleep, our brain is storing new information and processing toxic waste as our cells restore and repair nearly every function of the body. Sleep is critical to our well-being, which is why a healthy sleep environment is so important. Most mattresses contain flame retardants, rayon, fiberglass, boric acid, dyes, chemical adhesives such as polychloroprene, polyurethane foam that can emit VOCs or polyvinyl chloride (PVC), or vinyl covers that contain phthalates, fragrance chemicals, or conventional cotton that is often polluted with pesticides, herbicides, and fertilizers, or other undisclosed chemical treatments. Some suggest a correlation between the rise of sudden infant death syndrome (SIDS) and the application of flame-retardant compounds in mattresses.[36]

Opt for: *A mattress free of vinyl, polyurethane foam, added flame retardants, PFAS, antimicrobials, or added minerals*

AIR QUALITY

When indoors it's best to keep fresh air flowing as much as possible. Consider investing in a HEPA filter to minimize particulate matter and potential allergens to improve your indoor air quality.

Opt for: *Decals to decorate the nursery instead of painting. If painting indoors is unavoidable, choose VOC-free paints and plan to be out of the house for at least a few days to allow for the home to air out. Air plants make for sweet nursery décor and help purify air. If you have had any water intrusion issues or live in an older home, you may also want to consider testing your home for mold, asbestos, and lead.*

71

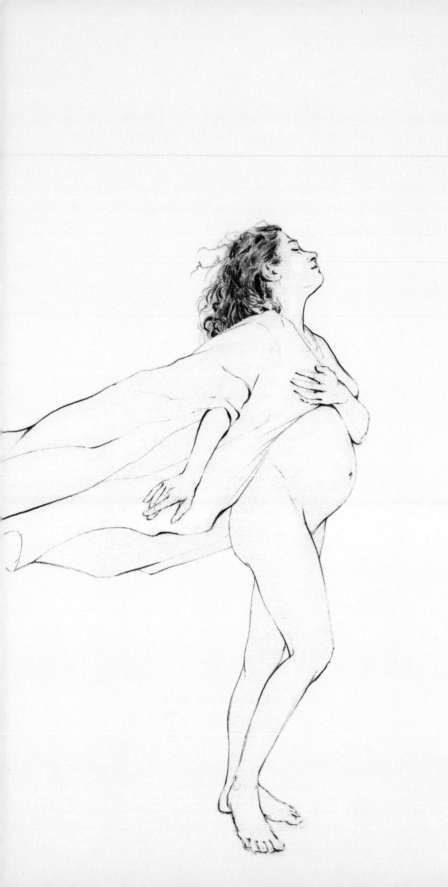

CELLULAR BIRTH MEMORIES

"We vibrate to the rhythms of our mother's blood
before she herself is born and this pulse is
the thread of blood that runs all the way back
through the grandmothers to the first mother."

LAYNE REDMOND

When my grandmother gave birth in the 1950s and '60s, a common labor practice was to give women a cocktail of anesthetic drugs called "twilight sleep." In *Birth: The Surprising History of How We Are Born*, Tina Cassidy describes strapping down their arms, "bandaging their eyes with gauze, and stuffing their ears to mask the sound of their own screams."[37] Rather than alleviating pain, twilight sleep just wiped one's memory of it, leaving a generation of women, like my grandmother, without birth stories to tell.

73

Years ago, when looking through old memorabilia, I came across a faded hospital card covered in Carnation formula images. This was the card given to my grandfather along with a cigar in the waiting room to let him know that his daughter had been born and was washed and ready to meet him in the nursery. In the late 1960s, only 15 percent of fathers were in the room when their child was born. At the time, breastfeeding was not a celebrated aspect of motherhood, and when I asked my grandmother if she knew anyone who breastfed she said, "Oh heavens, no! If they were, they certainly wouldn't do it in public nor talk about it."

Thirty years later, when my mother gave birth to me, many standard practices had changed for the better. Nationwide breastfeeding initiatives led to an increase in nursing rates, and although breastfeeding in public wouldn't be legal in all fifty states for another twenty-five years, the benefits were more widely recognized and embraced. By the 1990s, twilight sleep was long gone thanks to the introduction of the epidural and babies were encouraged to "room in" with their mothers instead of being sent off to nurseries where they were left untouched and alone.

However, progress is not always linear. In those thirty-three years, Cesarean rates rose from 4.5 percent to 23 percent and have increased another 10 percent since.[38] Today the maternal mortality rate is at its highest since 1965. The United States ranks among the highest in infant and maternal mortality rates in the developed world, falling behind Lebanon, the Gaza Strip, and Chile.[39] According to the National Institutes of Health, 45 percent of women experience traumatic childbirth.[40]

The overwhelming collective unease around childbirth makes perfect sense when we reflect on our recent history. How can women feel a sense of trust in the innate wisdom of the process and instill confidence in their daughters when they themselves have been demoralized? The experiences of the women who came before us are ingrained within our cells. Their fears, traumas, and resilience permeate through generations.

We have quite literally been carried by generations before us. We existed as an egg in our mother's ovaries while she was in the womb of our grandmother. Through the more recent exploration of epigenetics and how behaviors and the environment influence the way our genes work, science has caught up to the understanding that the lived experiences of our ancestors are stored within us and that through a deeper understanding of the original source of the trauma we can access greater resilience.

When my mother was induced at forty-two weeks pregnant, the room filled with visitors. My grandmother, my aunts, and my teenage sisters and their friends gathered around, each of them carrying with them their own lived experiences and programming around birth. My heart rate began to dip in response to the induction medication, and perhaps the environment, and she was instantly rushed into the operating room for a Cesarean; I was born shortly after. She doesn't remember much from the operating room except for staring into the "kind eyes" of a masked man who she later realized was my father.

I never thought much of my entrance until I became a doula and started to ask my mother more details about it. She told me she had read many books to prepare and wrote out her birth wishes; she wanted to practice yoga; have dim lighting, candles, and music; and be able to move around freely. In the moment no one really asked her what she wanted and instead she became the host of a welcome party, entertaining a room full of guests eagerly awaiting the newest member of our big, happy family. She recalls hiding in the bathroom to find moments of quiet and privacy during labor. She felt a pressure to perform. Knowing my mom, I'm sure it was hard for her, even in the midst of her birth, to step out of the role of a good wife, a nice stepmom, and an accommodating friend, sister, daughter, and patient and ask for what she needed: the space to birth. Perhaps on a subconscious level the operating room was where we ended up because it was relatively private.

Today my mother jokes, "Where were you when you were born?" What she longed for was a person who could hold space for the sacredness of birth, a doula. I have no doubt that my mother's birth experience with me planted the seed for the path I chose in life and shaped who I am today. In learning about and processing my arrival, it became clear to me that I was holding on to anxiety that didn't belong to me. I know my mother's birth experience propelled me to want to birth in a space of complete trust and to reclaim the intimacy she and I didn't get to have. I did not hesitate to put me, and my daughter's needs, above everyone else's and keep our birth space our own. Giving birth allowed me to heal and restore elements that were lost for the women who came before me, and it gave me the opportunity to reprogram what I had been led to believe about birth.

Fast forward to today, my daughter Lou is now 18 months old. I asked her recently, "Do you remember being born?" She nodded confidently. "What do you remember about it?" "Born in the bed," she said. She whipped her head back looking up to the sky, reenacting the exact position she was born in. "Mama did it! Dada caught me." This moment reenforced everything I knew to be true. She held a somatic memory of her birth.

Your Vantage Point

Spend some time this week reflecting on how the birth stories of the women who came before you shaped how you perceive pregnancy, birth, and motherhood today. If you're able, ask your mother what her experience was like, what feelings she recalls, what was going on in the world at the time, and whether she felt supported. Looking back through history, what has birth been like for the women in your lineage? Where might you be holding on to narratives that no longer serve you? How do you want your birth to feel different? How can you break free of old molds and conditioning around motherhood? What strength and wisdom from the women before you do you want to carry forth to the next generation?

RECONSIDERING ROUTINE ULTRASOUND

In the 1970s, ultrasound became a diagnostic tool for high-risk pregnancies, and in the fifty years since the machinery has evolved to create impressively clear 4D images that are now widely used in nearly all pregnancies regardless of risk factors. Ultrasounds are not only used as a medical diagnostic tool but are also marketed to parents recreationally as a means of bonding with their unborn child. There are boutiques popping up all over the country where expecting parents can pay to see their baby on the big screen. Some will even offer to come to your home where friends and family can take part in the experience for an additional fee.

This routinely utilized recreational and medical diagnostic tool used to peer inside the womb is often turned to as a means of alleviating concerns for parents and providers and has become somewhat of a rite of passage of pregnancy in the modern age. However, it is worth taking into consideration the potential drawbacks[41] that many parents are not informed of.

When my client Gwen went in for her anatomy scan at twenty weeks, she didn't think much of it. With zero risk factors or health concerns, she assumed this routine exam would leave her feeling confident in the health of her pregnancy and even more connected to her baby. After an hour scan, the well-regarded maternal-fetal medicine specialist had concerns that her baby's cerebellum was not developing and asked her to come back in two weeks so they could measure the growth. The follow-up ultrasound revealed that their baby's brain was growing as it should, but the doctor explained that there was a small benign cyst on her baby's brain and that it would likely dissolve on its own by twenty-eight weeks. They were asked to schedule another ultrasound just to be sure.

After the roller coaster of emotions she had been through, she was eager to have this final ultrasound to rule out any concerns once and for all. This time the doctor sat her down and told her that although the cyst had dissolved, this ultrasound revealed that one ventricle was measuring larger than the other and that this could be an indication of a severe abnormality and she may want to consider termination. He proceeded to offer her a prescription for Xanax and a referral to an MRI technician. The scan was intended to make her feel more confident and in control, but now she was overcome with worry.

"Deep down I knew he was healthy and just needed more time to fully develop, but it's hard to believe your gut instincts when a doctor is telling you otherwise. There were times I felt less connected to my baby as a result," Gwen said. After six hours of ultrasound testing over the span of two agonizing months, Gwen and her husband sought out a second opinion and prepared to greet their baby with loving arms

79

no matter what the diagnosis. The final ultrasound showed no concern, and she went on to give birth to a beautiful, healthy baby boy.

Over the years, I have seen ultrasound inaccuracies arise when analyzing fetal size, placenta health and placement, fluid levels, and even some serious developmental health concerns. The findings from ultrasounds often inform the route of birth. When concerns such as "big baby," calcified placenta, low fluid levels, and fetal growth restriction are detected, interventions such as early inductions and Cesareans are recommended. These interventions are not without risks. One would hope that the use of ultrasound technology would lead to improved birth outcomes, but even with the wide use of ultrasound today, the United States still ranks the highest in maternal and fetal deaths in the developed world.[42]

Given the limited safety studies, I didn't feel comfortable utilizing ultrasound to confirm my pregnancy when I knew it didn't guarantee a lasting one. At twenty weeks we decided to do a very brief ultrasound to look at our baby's major organs to be prepared to thoughtfully face any medical needs after birth. I understood the results of the ultrasound could be inaccurate and leave me with a false sense of security or unnecessary worry. There are many medical issues that can manifest throughout one's life, and an ultrasound is just a snapshot in time with great limitations. I also knew that routine ultrasound in a low-risk pregnancy is not an intervention that correlates with improved outcomes[43] or a guarantee of a healthy baby, every parent's greatest wish.

At our twenty-week scan I told the doctor that we did not want to know our baby's estimated weight or sex. I explained to him that I had concerns about ultrasound exposure and its implications on the baby and that I would like him to limit the ultrasound to two minutes. The doctor respectfully agreed but was quick to tell me that I had no reason to think the ultrasound would be in any way disruptive to my baby. As soon as the wand was placed on my belly, I felt a big wiggle. "Oh! Baby just flipped upside down," he said. It was all the confirmation I needed that she could in fact detect the pulsing sound waves.

When the sound waves of an ultrasound machine meet the tissue, bones, and fluid of the baby, the waves then bounce back and convert into an image on a screen. Studies have found that fetal movement increases with exposure to ultrasound and that children who had been exposed to ultrasound more frequently during pregnancy took longer to speak.[44] It has been documented that the children of mothers who were exposed to ultrasound were more likely to be left-handed as adults[45] and that ultrasound can damage the myelin that surrounds nerves in newborn rats. We don't know the significance of these findings, but one could infer that the brain and nervous system are susceptible to ultrasound exposure. Sonograms today have eight times the intensity of sound waves than prior to 1991 and the implications of that are not well studied.

As you approach week twelve and the routine scans or diagnostic tests offered to you at this stage, refer back to the road map questions from Week 8 to check in with yourself. Ask yourself how this tool and the information gained may impact your pregnancy. What are the benefits and risk and how do they pertain to you? Remember that just because something is routine does not mean it is mandatory. You get to choose how and when you utilize interventions to benefit your pregnancy.

Grounding Through Mother Earth

Over time, people have become more and more detached from the healing properties of Earth. We no longer sleep on the ground or walk barefoot outdoors. We spend most of our time indoors insulated from the fresh air, sunshine, and Mother Earth's biome. Several studies have confirmed what most of us already know to be true: touching our skin to the Earth decreases inflammation, lowers cortisol levels, and promotes healing.[46]

This week I invite you to get outside and plant your bare feet in the soil. As you soak in the medicine Mother Earth has to offer, release into the ground that which no longer serves you. Let any negativity you are carrying drain out of you and into the soil, where it can be transmuted by the restorative nature of Mother Earth.

EYE OF THE TIGER

At twelve weeks, nearly all your baby's organs are formed and continue to grow and develop each day. If you haven't already shared the news widely you may be feeling more ready now. For many the twelve-week mark comes with a feeling of relief because miscarriage rates drop by 80 percent this week. It is not uncommon for anxious feelings to persist, especially for mamas who have experienced pregnancy loss or fertility struggles. It's important to know that you are not alone in these feelings, and it is possible to transcend fear and relish the present moment.

Fear is defined as unpleasant emotion caused by the belief that someone or something is dangerous, likely to cause pain, or a threat. I want to point out an important key word: *belief*. Many of the worries that keep us up at night are not current threats but rather the anticipation of a nonexistent threat. Yet, this doesn't make them feel any less real.

In order to understand the purpose and impact of the stress response, picture a mama deer giving birth in the wild when all of a sudden she

83

hears rustling in the bushes. A hungry tiger is approaching. She senses danger and a rush of adrenaline pulses through her so she can fight or flee. Giving birth to a vulnerable baby covered in blood, followed by a placenta, in the presence of a tiger would not pan out well. This stress response stops the flow of hormones that produce contractions, allowing the deer to run to safety, where she can continue to labor. Humans are no different; when we are faced with the threat of danger, we release hormones that help us act as needed and get to safety. This is an example of a healthy stress response. In nature we see this stress response cycle through to its end so that the animal can carry on. Have you ever seen a dog shake after an unpleasant event? They are literally shaking off a traumatic or stressful experience.

Many of us live in a state of elevated stress even when we are not actually faced with the present threat of danger, but our bodies don't know the difference. This is the fear that serves no benefit. When we are in a constant state of hyperarousal and don't allow these feelings to flow through and out of us, it becomes more challenging to function optimally, make decisions from a centered place, and feel at home in our bodies.

An actual four-legged tiger is probably not going to show up at your doorstep, but "tigers" come in many different forms. Sometimes we bring them with us (anxious thoughts or past experiences), sometimes other people bring them into the space, and sometimes we do in fact have to come face-to-face with the tiger we so desperately want to avoid. These tigers often end up becoming our greatest teachers.

Noticing how our cognitive tigers affect our physical behavior is a key step in regulating anxiety. If a tiger presents itself, look the tiger in the eye, reminding yourself there is no tiger too big to tackle. With the proper support and tools, you are strong enough to face any tiger.

Get to Know Your "Tigers"

Oftentimes just acknowledging your fears and talking about them with your partner, your doula, or a specialist can help bring them to the surface so you can move through them. I find somatic therapy to be especially beneficial, and we will explore this modality more in a later section. Sharing our tigers makes us feel less alone and more equipped to respond. The medicine of connection should never be underestimated.

GET CLEAR ON YOUR TIGERS BY ASKING YOURSELF

- What are my tigers?

- Where are these tigers coming from? Are they mine, or are they someone else's? Is it possible I am picking up on my partner's tigers or my provider's tigers? Pregnancy is a particularly perceptive time, and it is possible to mistake other people's anxiety as our own. Take inventory of the external messages you receive from the outside world.

- Am I currently standing in front of this tiger or am I anticipating its presence?

- What does it feel like in my body?

- What are some ways I have overcome tigers in the past?

- How can I set myself up for support to feel confident facing whatever tigers I may encounter?

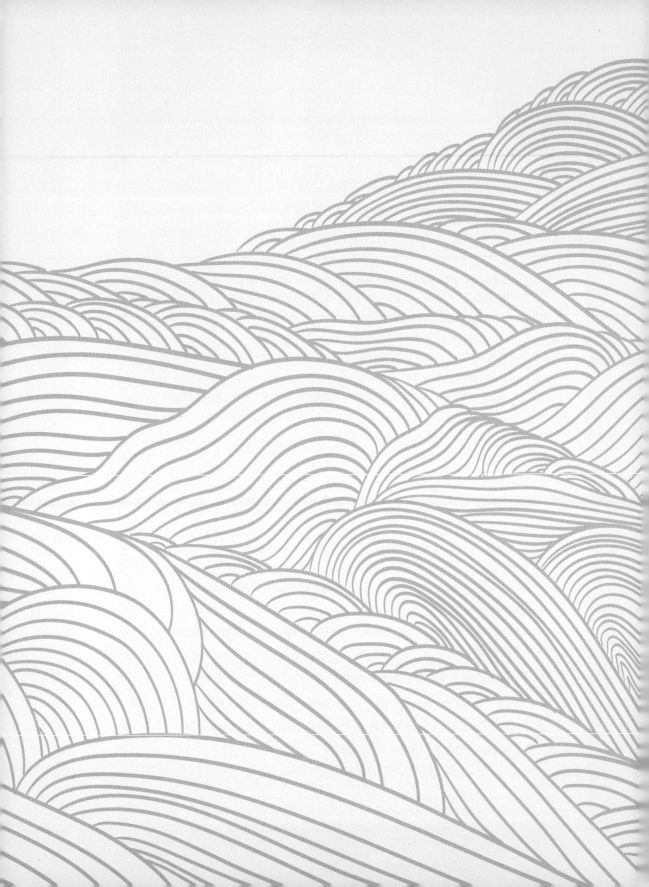

SECOND TRIMESTER

"Childbirth takes place at the intersection
of time; in all cultures it links past, present, and
future. In traditional cultures birth unites the world
of 'now' with the world of the ancestors and is
part of the great tree of life extending
in time and eternity."

SHEILA KITZINGER

VOICING YOUR POWER

Although you still have a ways to go until you get to hear the sweet sounds your baby will make, this week his vocal chords are developing in preparation for voicing his needs. We are hardwired to communicate freely from our very first breath and to be met with connection. Pregnancy is a potent time to reconnect with the innate connection to our throat chakra to prepare ourselves to voice our power freely for birth and motherhood.

So many of us were conditioned from a very first breath to be quiet. Most of us have been shushed, pacified, and left to cry alone in our most formative years, which ingrains the message that children should grow to "be seen and not heard." How our parents responded to our cries as a baby shaped how we communicate today. How we respond to our children's needs is intrinsically linked with how comfortable we are with voicing our own. For some of us we may be able to pinpoint when exactly in our lives we were shut down or told to be quiet, and for others it may be traced back through a lineage that experienced oppression and silencing.

The throat chakra is connected to your ability to communicate and speak your inner truth. Our throat chakras are located just behind the thyroid glands at the base of the neck. This area is intrinsically linked to the pelvis. The word *cervix* is the Latin word for "neck" of the uterus. As embryos, the throat and womb grow side by side before eventually moving away from one another. You can see here that there are similarities in structure, and both are held by a hammock-like set of diaphragmatic muscles that move in conjunction with the breath. When we tense the jaw, our pelvic floor follows suit. When we relax and release the jaw, we allow for release.

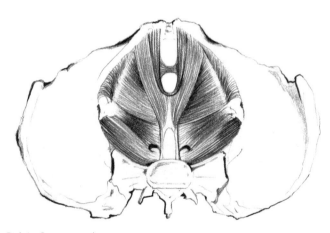

Pelvic floor muscles

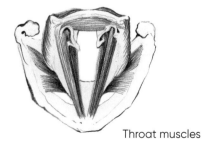

Throat muscles

You may have seen birth videos of animals or women moaning or making "om" sounds in labor. These primal low-register sounds are quite literally working in harmony with the pelvic floor. Birth is loud, primal, messy, and fierce. It's BIG work. It's heaven and hell, birth and death all in one, and it's the most profoundly intense experience. There is nothing tidy, timid, or polite about it. For generations women have been conditioned to be small, not to take up too much space, and mocked for feeling the full extent of their emotions. As women, we're often expected to be quiet and nice and not scare anyone with our intensity and magnitude. Birth can shatter that. It invites you to unleash those chains if you want to.

I have been a witness to ecstatic births that were completely silent, and I have watched mothers roar their children into the world with power and ecstasy, both with and without medication. For me, screaming was the only way I could make it through the portal. With each howl I felt I was calling her earthside. It grounded me. It matched my strength in volume. It allowed me to unleash and feel completely embodied. I didn't want to be numb to it. I thought I would be a quiet birther, but I screamed for hours and hours. In between my screams I spoke to my daughter. I praised her. Told her I loved her and made sure she knew I was not screaming at her. I wanted her to hear me be loud in my power so she can always feel safe to express hers.

●

AFFIRMATION INSPIRATION

I feel and express the magnitude of my experience with courage.
I am safe to speak my truth.
My voice is worthy of being heard.

Unleash the Throat Chakra

This week's activity includes both inner and outer work to deepen the connection to your power and voicing your needs.

PART ONE • JOURNALING QUESTIONS

- Where in my lineage have my ancestors been silenced?

- Where did I learn that I could get myself into trouble if I used my voice?

- What is the worst that would happen if I spoke my truth?

- How comfortable am I voicing my needs?

- Do I feel obligated to follow directives from authority figures even if it goes against my needs?

- Where in my life am I holding back from speaking my truth?

PART TWO • VOCAL EXERCISES

Part two of this exercise is to put your power into practice. One of the simplest and most effective ways to connect to your throat chakra is by using your voice. Perhaps this means getting something off your chest and finding the courage to voice your needs. This could also look like singing at the top of your lungs each day in the shower, chanting as a daily meditation practice, or repeating your own personal affirmation out loud.

NUTRIENTS TO CONSIDER IN THE SECOND TRIMESTER

By week fourteen most women start to feel their appetite return and nausea subside. This is a great time to focus on replenishing and building nutrients for your growing baby and in preparation for optimal health in the postpartum period.

Iron: Optimal iron levels are important for fetal and maternal health, and deficiency has been linked to preterm birth and delayed cognitive development in babies. During pregnancy, your blood volume increases by 40 to 50 percent, which necessitates more iron-rich foods. For mothers, symptoms of low iron can include fatigue, depression, and anxiety. When building iron stores, the focus should always be on incorporating bioavailable food. The most commonly used iron supplements are ferrous fumarate and ferrous sulfate.[47] However, 45 percent of people experience unpleasant side effects such as constipation, nausea, heartburn, and stomach pain as a result of these forms of iron. Although iron can be found in plant foods, these non-heme sources are significantly less absorbable than heme sources of iron, which is why I believe red meat is an essential food for pregnancy. • Where to find it: *Beef, liver, shellfish, poultry, lentils*

Calcium: With the rapid growth of your baby's skeletal system, calcium needs increase. Midway through the second trimester at around twenty weeks calcium needs double to support baby's growing bones! Since this is such an important task, regardless of the amount of calcium mom consumes, your baby will prioritize getting enough by pulling from your stores. Replenishing your reserves is essential for maintaining your bone health and ensuring you have adequate calcium for the milk you will soon be making. If you do not consume dairy on a regular basis, additional supplementation may be necessary. • Where to find it: *Cow, goat, and sheep milk, sardines, sesame seeds*

B12: Vitamin B12 is involved in the synthesis of DNA and red blood cells. Deficiency can result in fatigue, lethargy, and weakness as well as anxiety and depression during and after pregnancy. B12 is most abundant in animal products. • Where to find it: *Organ meats, salmon, cottage cheese*

SKIN FOOD

Pregnancy can come with greater sensitivity to the sun and the formation of skin tags, dark spots, acne, and, of course, stretch marks. Your

93

susceptibility to stretch marks depends on the elasticity of your skin. To promote skin elasticity, you will want to prioritize ample moisture from naturally derived topical ingredients such as tallow, shea butter, sea buckthorn, and jojoba oil.

It is equally important to nourish and hydrate your skin from the inside out with foods rich in amino acids such as glycine and collagen. Glycine and collagen can be found in bone broth, organ meats, and fish. Foods containing vitamin C (broccoli, camu camu, jujube, green bell pepper, and fruits) will help your body synthesize collagen. Vitamin C supports iron absorption and a healthy immune system. It also aids in the production of collagen for greater skin elasticity and may promote a strong amniotic sac.

Vitamin C Jujube Elixir

Rich in vitamin C antioxidants, this tea is hydrating, helps with circulation, and can be added to soups for a deliciously sweet taste.

1 cup [200 g] organic dried jujubes
Organic ginger root
Organic dried goji berries

Pit and roughly chop the jujubes. Leaving the skin on, slice the ginger into ½ in [1.3 cm] thick slices. Place the jujubes and ginger in a large pot with 2 qt water over medium-high heat and add the goji berries to taste. Bring to a simmer and cook for 30 minutes, adding more water as needed to taste.

Drink as desired for hydration and immunity support. Can be stored in a mason jar in the fridge and enjoyed cold or reheated.

THE MATERNAL MICROBIOME

Our babies inherit our microbiome through pregnancy, birth, skin-to-skin contact, and breastfeeding,[48] which is reason to prioritize beneficial bacteria through probiotic-rich foods, spending more time in nature, avoiding antibiotics, minimizing environmental toxins, and reducing inflammation through healthy lifestyle choices. By populating your microbiome with beneficial bacteria, you are supporting your newborn's immune system and digestion, and lowering their risk of allergies, asthma, thrush, and eczema.

Probiotic-rich foods are important for populating your gut with healthy bacteria that can help you ward off infection and aid in absorption and digestion of foods. Additionally, sour foods help curb sugar cravings, which makes fermented foods a great snack. Fermented foods include kefir, kombucha, pickled veggies, sauerkraut, kimchi, and natto. These can be found in the refrigerator aisle of the grocery store and should not be mistaken for vinegar brine pickled veggies.

Creating Healthy Habits

Your nutritional choices today have a big influence on your baby's health and development. Once your baby is earthside, she will continue to lean on you for nutrients and guidance. Our children learn by example.

This week, take note of what healthy habits you want to incorporate into your life to be a positive role model for your baby. What healthy habits do you want your child to observe?

Take your commitment to nourishment one step further and participate in the production and preparation of food however you can. This is a beautiful way to connect with the creative energy and gifts of Mother Nature. This could look like starting a garden, having a window box of herbs, getting a chicken coop, composting, or even just spending more time preparing home-cooked meals with food from your local farmers' market.

INTENTIONAL MOVEMENT

Now that you are in the second trimester you may be getting some of your energy back and feeling those early pregnancy symptoms a bit less. If you've engaged in little physical activity over the past couple of months, you're not alone. Now is a great time to get into a flow of intentional daily movement that will support your growing body and baby in preparation for birth and beyond.

People are often quick to state the "do's and don'ts" of exercise in pregnancy, but you are the expert on you and I wholeheartedly believe that when you listen to your body you will know what exercises you should avoid. I can't emphasize enough that when exercising in pregnancy you should never disregard discomfort or pain nor minimize any physical messages from your body. As women, we have been conditioned to hold our bellies in tight for flat abs and to overexert ourselves to achieve a "desirable" physique. Exercise in pregnancy should be done strictly to feel good mentally and physically, as an act of service, love,

97

and acceptance toward your body and baby. Whatever physical activity you engage in should not deplete you or overly tighten you but rather leave you feeling more energized and comfortable. Yoga, swimming, walking, stretching, and belly dancing are wonderful ways to reap the benefits of movement with low impact and risk of injury.

Regardless of how you incorporate movement into your day, understanding the pelvic floor is key. The pelvic floor is a set of muscles and connective tissue located at the base of the pelvis. This hammock-like group of muscles supports the organs above it and is a part of the core muscles that stabilize the spine.

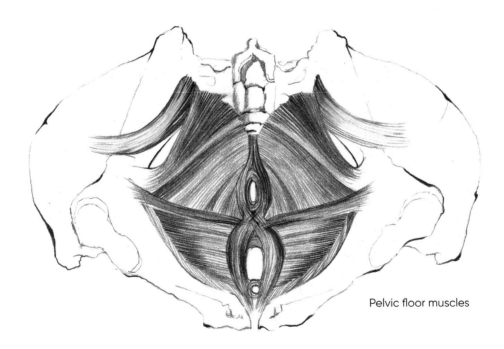

Pelvic floor muscles

The ABCs of the Pelvic Floor

This week's activity is from Allison Oswald, Los Angeles's go-to pelvic floor therapist. Her support was so valuable to me in pregnancy and early motherhood. Here Allison will walk you through the pelvic floor ABCs to help you create a mindful awareness of your pelvic floor muscles in preparation for pregnancy and the postpartum period.

FROM ALLISON

Prenatal pelvic floor work is all about developing a deeper connection to the inner core, which can help alleviate incontinences, constipation, low back pain, and sexual discomfort while preparing the body for birth and the postpartum period.

All too often pregnancy and postpartum discomforts are brushed off as common and expected aspects of the journey. Just because something is common does not mean it's normal, and there is so much you can do to support your pelvic floor to feel your best. As you exercise, walk, sit at your desk, stretch, or simply move about your day, experiment with these tips to support your connection with your pelvic floor.

A • ALIGNMENT

Standing or sitting, try to keep your rib cage over your pelvis comfortably without overarching or rounding your low back. This is not a rigid stance, but a good rule of thumb is to feel like the weight of your body is evenly distributed between both feet, as well as the balls and heels of the feet, when you're standing.

When sitting, be sure
to sit on your sitz bones. This alignment can
give you better access to your deep core as well
as put less pressure on the pelvic floor.

B • BREATHING

Imagine your diaphragm at the base of your rib cage being the top
of your core and the pelvic floor being the bottom of the core. You
want to start with sitting where those two are parallel as explained
in the alignment section. Then inhale, feeling your rib cage expand
360 degrees (not up into your shoulders or neck). As this is happening,
the diaphragm is expanding down, and the pelvic floor is too. As
you exhale, the diaphragm recoils up as the rib cage comes back in
and the pelvic floor moves up as well. This diaphragmatic breathing
practice improves pelvic floor function along with so many other
benefits, such as calming your nervous system, aiding in digestion,
improving blood flow, and coordinating the deepest core movements.

C • CONNECTION

As you learned in the breathing section, the pelvic floor moves
up (contracts) with the exhale. So now, you can begin to use
the exhale during activities or movements when you need more
support because when you exhale you are activating your
pelvic floor a bit. Other daily tips are to always relax rather than
strain when you use the bathroom, move your body at least
twenty minutes every day, drink plenty of water, and work with
a pelvic floor therapist if concerns arise.

You may want to invest in a birth ball to sit on instead
of a desk chair or couch. Birth balls promote mobility in
the pelvis and can be a useful tool when exploring the
relationship between breath and your pelvic floor.

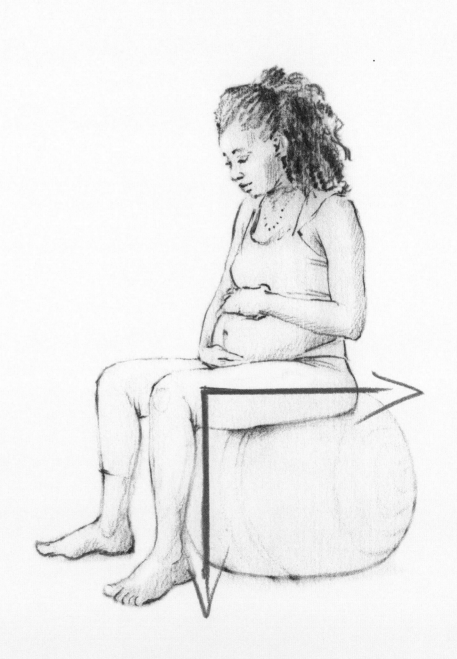

DROPPING OUT OF YOUR HEAD AND INTO YOUR BODY

By now some mamas have started to feel little kicks and squirms. These early wiggles can often be mistaken for gas, but soon they will undeniably be the squirming sensations of your baby! If your placenta is anterior (located in the front) it may take longer for you to feel your baby kick because the placenta acts as a pillow between your baby and the wall of your uterus. As you feel these sensations more, set aside time daily to tune into her rhythms, noticing the patterns and cadence of movement as she grows.

MOTHER NATURE'S WISDOM

During my pregnancy, springtime in my garden was more majestic to me than ever before. As I planted seeds and patiently waited for their readiness, I felt this process mirror the inner world inside me. How simple yet profound the creation of life, and how little we must do for it to happen. One afternoon while watering my plants, I saw a mother dove sitting in her nest tucked away in a pine tree. She too was waiting for her baby to hatch, and I remember feeling comforted by the fact that we were both growing life side by side in two very different ways. I knew that her innate maternal instincts were probably very similar to mine: to keep her young safe. Yet it wasn't lost on me that she wasn't consumed by external pressure or expectation for her chicks to hatch by a certain date or worried about how or where it should take place. I began to research mourning doves and learned that they mate for life, which I imagine is why they are a symbol for love. I also learned that both mom and dad doves build their nest together and share in the responsibility of incubating and feeding the chicks once they hatch.

We have so much to discover about birth from observing Mother Nature. When we watch animals birth it is a profound reminder that birth is not something we need to use our prefrontal cortex to do. In fact, it is easier to give birth when we drop out of our heads and into our bodies. Nobody instructs a wild animal how to give birth. They don't read pregnancy books, they don't concern themselves with self-doubt, and they don't question their ability to nurture and care for their young. They rely solely on their innate wisdom to bring life forward. The act of giving birth is a normal biological function and they know exactly how to birth and step into their role as a mother. Guess what . . . so do you!

Birth in the Wild

One of my favorite ways to support parents in preparation for birth is to have them observe animals giving birth in the wild. If you don't live among wildlife, you have access to endless videos on YouTube.

This week's activity is to watch animal birth videos and reflect on what you observe and how it may look similar to or different from your experience. How can you turn to the natural world to find more peace and deeper connection to your inner wisdom? How can the rhythms of nature help prepare you for motherhood?

TREE OF LIFE

You are well into your second trimester and nearly halfway to the finish line! Your umbilical cord is becoming longer, thicker, and stronger and is carrying oxygenated blood and nutrients to the placenta. There will come a time where feeding your baby takes effort, but for now, you're giving your baby all he needs to grow and thrive without any thought at all! The umbilical cord is symbolic of your innate ability to mother and the lifeblood that flows from you to your baby. Take a second to acknowledge that no one needs to tell you how or what to do for this process to happen seamlessly. All the wisdom is hardwired within you.

The umbilical cord and placenta are often referred to as the Tree of Life, not just because they are a vital component of life on Earth but also because of the unmistakable treelike structure formed from the arteries, veins, and umbilical cord.

When a baby is born she is still connected to her mother as long as the placenta remains inside the womb and the umbilical cord remains

105

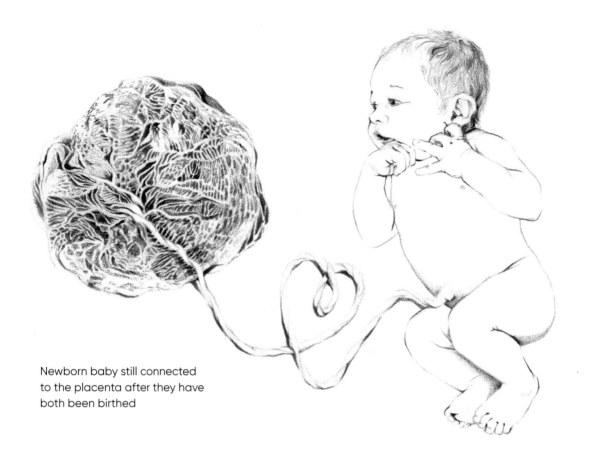

Newborn baby still connected
to the placenta after they have
both been birthed

intact. This is nature's way of telling us that although one has become two, it is vital that they stay close to one another. This cord tethers baby to her mother's body, the safest place for her to be. The umbilical cord continues to pulsate after the baby is born to help her transition to the world outside the womb and support her as she acclimates to a new method of oxygenation. Although babies practice breathing in utero, they don't breathe oxygen until they leave the aquatic environment they were in.

Over the past century with the medicalization of birth, it has become common practice to sever the cord immediately upon arrival. This intervention disregards nature's design of keeping mother and baby attached after birth, and we now know through research that it comes with consequences.

To approach birth with a reverence for its physiological design is to understand that the pulsing umbilical cord is still supporting baby while she's working to take her very first breath. Your baby's cord blood serves a purpose after birth and is delivering nearly one-third of a baby's blood volume from the placenta during this time.[49] The benefit of a pulsing cord unsevered after birth is not just to help oxygenate the baby. Research has found several benefits associated with delayed cord clamping, such as an increase in fine motor and social skills[50] and improved newborn iron levels for up to six months after birth.[51]

The term "delayed cord clamping" doesn't have an exact definition. Some providers consider delayed clamping to be a couple of minutes after birth, while others consider it the full transfusion of blood from the placenta to the baby. It is important to make the distinction when communicating with your provider. If you want to allow the cord to pulsate completely until all of the blood is transferred to the baby before clamping and cutting the cord, be sure to say just that. Some providers consider delayed clamping to be one or two minutes and there is no way of knowing how long a full transfusion of blood will take.

WHAT IF BABY HAS HIS CORD WRAPPED AROUND HIS NECK AT BIRTH?

A mucous connective tissue called Wharton's jelly protects the umbilical vessels so the fetus can move and turn without compression of his blood supply. Some hypothesize that a baby who wraps himself in his

107

cord in utero is actually doing so to keep the cord from prolapsing at birth, which can restrict blood flow to the baby.

Thirty percent of babies are born with a nuchal cord.[52] There is no evidence that a nuchal cord during labor results in short-term or long-term mortality or morbidity[53] and is not a medical reason for a Cesarean delivery. How a doctor or midwife approaches a nuchal cord is a key factor in the safety of delivery with a cord present. Cutting or clamping the cord before baby's body has emerged can lead to hypoxia or an increased need for resuscitation. This practice is not evidence based and has been deemed malpractice in judicial findings. Keeping the cord intact and unwrapping the baby after birth is going to allow for optimal oxygenation and blood flow to the baby.

SHOULD I BANK MY BABY'S CORD BLOOD?

With the emerging advancements of stem cell research there has been a lot of buzz around banking newborn cord blood and tissue for parents to have peace of mind and the potential to cure a life-threatening condition. Selling parents on the prospect of this technology is a big business that raked in over $18 billion in 2020 and is projected to grow to $45 billion by 2026. However, in the event that a baby needs such treatment, it is unlikely that his own cord blood would be used, as these cord blood stem cells would carry the same problematic precursor cells. Together, two of the largest private cord blood banks in the United States have collected over a million units, yet only a few hundred units of it has ever been used in transplants.[54] Healthy donor blood seems to be of more value than one's own private reserve.

What is often left out of the conversation is that banking cord blood stops your baby from receiving the complete transfusion at birth and the benefits that come with it. The choice is personal, and the ever-evolving landscape of medical research may unlock greater advancements that make this a more worthwhile investment for your child in the future. A question to consider when weighing your options is, is it a person's birthright to receive their blood and stem cells at birth?

HONORING THE PLACENTA

When we look to nature, we find that nearly every mammal eats their placenta after birth. We don't know exactly why, but it is likely done to hide the smell of blood and keep hungry predators away. There is little research available on the benefits of humans consuming their placentas, but many mothers and birth workers observe an increase in energy, breast milk production, and mood stabilization with placenta consumption. It is possible that this is due to the iron, oxytocin, and lactogen contained in the placenta. It has been utilized medicinally in traditional Chinese medicine for thousands of years.[55]

Placentophagy is also utilized as a method by midwives for suppressing postpartum hemorrhaging.[56] Though there are not any studies done on this, the fact that placentas contain blood-clotting particles in addition to oxytocin points to their effectiveness in potentially helping to stop bleeding after birth. Midwives have found that putting a bit of placenta membrane in a mother's mouth or having her suck on the cord or a small quarter-size piece of placenta immediately helps manage blood loss.

If you are on the fence about placental encapsulation (transforming the placenta into pills), you can always preserve your placenta and then wait and see how you feel after giving birth. I lost very little blood, had plenty of breast milk and energy, and did not feel it was necessary for me to utilize the pills, although I had planned to. I was glad to have the option available to me as a remedy if the need arose, but ultimately I didn't feel drawn to taking them.

109

Regardless of whether you plan to consume your placenta or not, your placenta doesn't have to become medical waste. In many cultures the placenta is considered to be a guardian angel that connects the child to the spirit of his ancestors. Burying the placenta is believed to bestow blessings of protection for the child's future.

WAYS TO UTILIZE YOUR PLACENTA

Tincture: This gives it the longest life span.

Dehydrated and encapsulated: This can be done at home or by a doula, midwife, or placenta encapsulation company.

Raw blended in a smoothie: Some choose to consume their placenta raw by blending it into a smoothie.

Placenta print: Placing your placenta on a large white paper will make a beautiful Tree of Life keepsake print.

Dried umbilical cord: When our doula encapsulated my placenta she dried out the umbilical cord in the shape of a heart as a memento.

Planting a tree: If you don't plan to consume your placenta, you can bury it under a planted tree, which in Japanese and Chinese cultures is believed to bestow protection over the child. Planting a tree together is a beautiful way to honor the interconnectedness of all beings.

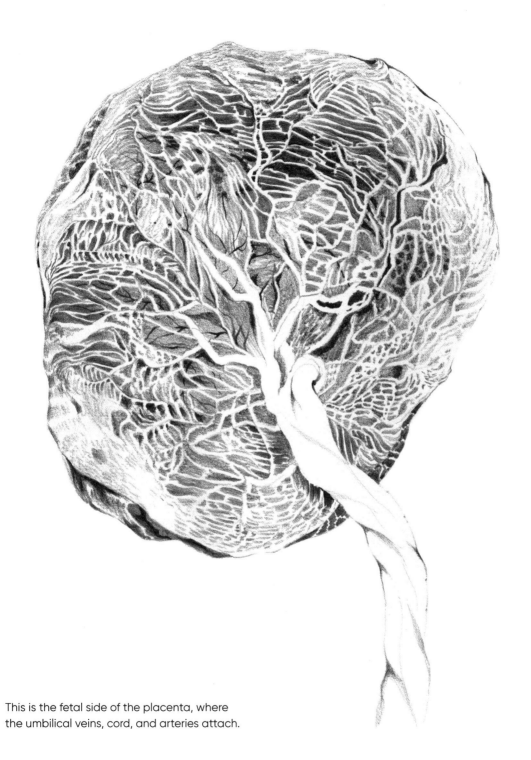

This is the fetal side of the placenta, where
the umbilical veins, cord, and arteries attach.

The Cosmic Connection Meditation

Place your hands over your womb space on each side of your belly button and take a few slow, deep breaths to ground yourself and quiet the chatter in your mind. Bring your awareness to your belly button located between your solar plexus and sacral chakra. The belly button is the portal where you once received nourishment and oxygen from your mother. For just a moment, put aside whatever complexities exist in your relationship with your mother today and appreciate the life force that poured from her to you and now allows you to do the same for your child.

Visualize your baby in your womb, warm, cozy, and soothed by the rhythm of your heart and the cadence of your breath. With each slow and deep inhale and exhale, see a growing light radiating from your solar plexus all around your belly and expanding around your entire body, creating an orb of light. This orb exists as your amniotic sac, just like your baby's. It is your own protective space that you can access any time you need to. It is a place of peace and serenity. There is space for you to move and stretch around while feeling the warm, strong, and snug support of being held and carried.

Now imagine there is an umbilical cord that reaches from the
top of this sac up into the sky, past the clouds and Earth's
atmosphere and into the cosmos. Perhaps it is connected
to the sun, the moon, a star, a guardian angel, or God.
Whatever the source may be, feel the all-consuming warmth
of unconditional love and protection that it delivers to you.

Tuning in to the pulsing cord that connects from
your baby's belly button to your placenta, send
that same feeling of protection and any messages
of love through the cord and to your baby.

*For an audio recording of this meditation
visit my website www.carson-meyer.com.*

THE RHYTHM OF LOVE

By eighteen weeks, your baby's ears can pick up some sound in the womb like your heartbeat, and her ability to hear and distinguish voices will advance in the coming weeks. Several studies have found that newborn infants remember sounds, melodies, and rhythmic poems they have been exposed to during fetal life and that exposure to music can have long-term impact on the developing brain. Knowing this, Johnathan and I created a nightly ritual of playing the guitar and singing to Lou in my belly. This practice was as much for us as it was for her.

CONNECTION AND COMMUNICATION
FOR CO-REGULATION

It is well documented that stress impacts a developing fetus and can have negative implications on lifelong mental and immunological health. In a perfect world every pregnant mother is immune from all stressors, but we know that's just not the reality for most people. Life happens, and trying to shield yourself and your baby from any and all stress is just not realistic. I hope it brings you some solace to know that some stress is actually associated with greater heart rate variability that helps prepare your baby for the outside world. Stress is unavoidable; it's how you repair and recover that matters most to promote peace for you and your baby. Every hurdle presents an opportunity to lay a foundation for open communication and model the tools you want to pass down so that one day your baby can confidently navigate whatever comes her way.

The nervous system of one individual influences another individual through a phenomenon called co-regulation. Social connection is a key factor in quieting the physiological stress responses at any age, but from pregnancy through the first three years of life, babies rely on our nervous system to regulate. Co-regulation is the reason why social connection is so important for our well-being. Connection activates regions in the brain that detect safety and inhibit physiological stress responses when they are not needed.

Whenever conflict, worry, or pressure arose in me I talked to Lou about it (sometimes out loud and sometimes just mentally). I explained to her that we are safe, that none of my feelings of stress had anything to do with her. I told her that I am strong and capable of navigating whatever comes our way and that sometimes feeling big emotions is just part of life. This established a connection between us that I used throughout my labor and every day since. It granted me the opportunity to be patient with myself and others and to create a framework for me to parent with.

Baby Talk

Carve out some time every day to talk to your baby, sing a song, or read him a book. Knowing that your baby is listening, how can you shift the way you speak about yourself and/or others in your life to model kindness and healthy communication?

FILL YOUR CUP

You are about to enter a season of life where the structure of your day no longer revolves around just your needs. The changing pace of parenthood makes it challenging to slow down and carve out intentional time to fill your cup. Pregnancy is not a time to pack it all in and grind to the finish line. It is a time to actively practice slowing down, to relish in your independence and create meaningful rituals that you can carry with you into motherhood. Ritual doesn't mean obsessing over doing something at the same time every day and shouldn't feel like a chore. How you incorporate ritual into your life for deeper connection and flow is personal.

We all have daily rituals and rhythms whether we realize it or not. They can be as simple as making a cup of coffee every morning, reading a few pages of a book before bed, or saying your prayers each night. Maybe you meditate daily or walk your dog before heading to work. Think about the daily rituals that you want to leave behind in parenthood and the ones you want to prioritize.

A DAILY MINDFUL MEDITATION

Get comfortable lying down or in a seated position. Place your hands on your womb and take three deep belly breaths. Feel your seat planted on the surface beneath you and visualize roots stemming from the bottom of your feet down through the floor, the foundation of your home, through the soil and bedrock. See these roots wrapping around Mother Earth. Feel how her strength stabilizes you. No matter how windy it is on the surface, you're being held steady by her soil.

Bringing your attention back to your womb, notice how with each deep breath the space around your baby grows and with each exhale your baby feels an embrace. Your diaphragm is located right above your uterus, and each inhale and exhale is a rhythmic dance communicating to your baby. When you slow and deepen your breath, you are demonstrating to your baby the type of breath that delivers deep relaxation to the nervous system.

Place one hand over your heart to tune in to the rhythm of its beat. Notice whether it's beating fast or slow. Perhaps you can take a few nice slow, deep breaths to help slow your heart rate for further relaxation. With one hand on your belly and one hand over your heart, feel the synchronicity of the two heartbeats within you.

For an audio recording of this meditation
visit my website www.carson-meyer.com.

Create an Altar

Create an altar with objects of meaning where you can go to meditate, pray, journal, or just sit quietly for five minutes each day to reflect and connect with your baby. My altar held written affirmations, candles, collected objects from nature, and photos. When it came time to give birth we positioned the birth tub in front of the altar. If you are birthing in a hospital or birth center, you can bring some altar items with you to hold on to wherever you are.

Week 20

YOUR RIPENING BODY

The half(ish) way mark is here! You are probably feeling those strong kicks and wiggles right about now. Your baby is practicing the sucking reflex and is now covered in vernix to protect her skin from pruning up in the amniotic environment. Some women start to feel "Braxton-Hicks" contractions in the second trimester. I prefer to call them practice contractions because (a) why should we title a strictly female sensation after a male doctor who claims to have discovered something women have been feeling since the beginning of time and (b) that is precisely what they are, practice contractions. Your uterine muscles are working out and warming up for their impending Olympic event. If these contractions seem stronger than usual sometimes the body is trying to signal the need for more downtime. Proper hydration and a magnesium salt bath should do the trick.

For some women the second trimester comes with a heightened libido and stronger orgasms. The fullness of your ripening body may have you feeling extra sensual as your energy increases in the second trimester. On the other hand it is common and completely normal for sex to be the last thing on your mind.

Once Johnathan was able to feel our baby's kicks from the outside, I sensed reticence from him around sex. Even though I reassured him that it was not going to hurt our baby, there was a mental hurdle for him that, at times, left me feeling rejected. As I got bigger and bigger it became more challenging to find comfortable or pleasurable positions for both of us. "If I am being completely honest," he said to me, "it feels like I am having sex with a bowling ball." We broke out in tears of laughter and I told him that would go down in history as one of the top ten worst things to say to your pregnant partner. With patience, communication, and creativity, we were able to find our rhythm again.

Pregnancy sex has myriad health benefits like stress relief and pelvic floor engagement. Some research has suggested that exposure to semen in pregnancy can decrease the likelihood of preeclampsia.[57] Your baby is well insulated behind the cervix and the amniotic fluid acts as a protective barrier. There is no reason to abstain from intercourse if you don't want to. Honor where you're at. There are many ways to stay connected and deepen intimacy with your partner as your lovemaking evolves. Challenge yourself to transform discomfort, awkwardness, or feelings of rejection into moments of deeper vulnerability and curiosity. Release expectation and be present in the process.

Red Raspberry, Nettle, and Oat Straw Infusion

Red raspberry leaf is one of the most widely used herbs in pregnancy and has a long history of traditional use to help tonify the uterus. It has been linked to a reduced likelihood of Cesarean, preterm or post-term labor, and may even shorten labor. Nettle is a mineral-rich herb high in vitamin K to support bone health and reduce inflammation, manage blood sugar, and alleviate allergies. Oat straw is soothing to the nervous system. I drank this infusion daily throughout pregnancy.

2 Tbsp organic red raspberry leaf
2 Tbsp organic dried stinging nettles
1 tsp organic oat straw
2 cups [480 ml] water

Place the herbs into a 1 qt [1 L] mason jar or French press. Bring the water to a boil and pour over the herbs. Steep for at least 20 minutes. Strain and drink 1 to 2 cups [240 to 480 ml] daily.

123

Writing Your Love Story

"Making love" really takes on an entirely new meaning in pregnancy. Together, you quite literally made love! Physical intimacy is the catalyst to this journey and emotional intimacy is an essential ingredient. This week I invite you to write a letter to your baby and share with her the love story of her parents. Tell her all the things you love about her father, what makes him an amazing partner, and what will make him a wonderful parent. This is an activity both of you can partake in. Share your letters with each other as a reminder of how far you've come together. File this away and revisit it with your partner after birth.

Week 21

HOME BIRTH

Hospital birth has only become the standard in the United States in the past hundred or so years. Although it is the norm, over the span of human history it is a relatively new phenomenon. Today, around 2 percent of women choose to give birth outside of the hospital, but the number has been increasing since 2004. According to a recent survey, there was a 22 percent increase in home births from 2019 to 2020[58] and has remained elevated since. The pandemic had an impact on many aspects of society, including work life, education, and even how we birth. People who had never entertained home birth prior were suddenly drawn to the idea of a peaceful and safe environment with the freedom to birth on their terms, with their desired support, outside of a broken health care system.

Of course, home birth isn't going to be the right choice for everyone. Although 85 percent of women are considered low risk and eligible for home birth, many women prefer to utilize the epidural, which is not offered at home. Over the years I have supported families both at home and in the hospital and I believe that the best place to birth is the place you feel the safest and are able to have access to the support and tools you desire. For me there was no question: home was where I wanted to be. These are some of the factors that influenced my choice to birth at home.

WHY I CHOSE TO BIRTH AT HOME

In the comfort of my own home, I was free to labor and birth without the limitations of hospital policies. I knew it was the atmosphere where my mind and body would be able to drop into the birthing process uninterrupted, allowing the physiological process to unfold safely. I knew that my likelihood of having a Cesarean would be lower at home. The Cesarean rate for planned home birth is as low as 6 percent, and this is five times lower than the national average.

Unless indicated otherwise, I don't perceive birth to be an emergency or medical ailment but instead a healthy function of the female body. Hospitals and surgeons play a crucial role treating emergency situations, but in no other time in my life would I seek out their support in the absence of a medical emergency. To me, birth is no exception.

Maternal satisfaction is higher in a home birth setting.

Feeling the full extent of birth was an important part of the process for me. I knew that I would have more freedom of movement and comfort at home.

I understand that there is no such thing as a risk-free birth regardless of location and circumstance. I am not under the illusion that choosing a hospital birth guarantees safety for me or my baby. A vast majority of births in the United States take place in the hospital and yet we have the highest maternal mortality rate of the developed world. We can be met with the unexpected regardless of where we birth.

126

Get Inspired

When I shared my birth story on social media, hundreds of expecting mothers wrote to tell me that reading my story expanded their beliefs about birth and inspired them to make empowered choices for themselves. For some, this meant pivoting to home birth, and for others it meant advocating for their birth choices within the hospital setting. Social media certainly has its drawbacks, but one of the gifts it can afford us is giving us access to different perspectives that inspire us.

My friend Lacy Philips works as a manifestation expert and is the founder of To Be Magnetic. She coined the term "Expander" to describe the people who help expand your belief system in a positive way. She writes, "What inspires us about others is a mirror of our capacity and capability. Therefore, when we watch a movie and get entranced by an actor, or a character in a book, or obsess over a public figure, or on social media, or someone that we admire in our daily lives, we are actually recognizing aspects of ourselves (denied or unmet) that have yet to integrate, and they are inviting us to grow into them. We are witnessing our potential greater than where we currently are, and where we are capable of going."

This week I invite you to meditate on your mama Expanders. Who do you admire as a parent and why? What kind of energy do they bring to parenthood and how do you want to integrate this quality to bring you closer to your authentic mama self in pregnancy, birth, and beyond?

Week 22

PROTECTING YOUR ENERGY FIELD

Now that you're well into the second trimester, chances are your sweet baby bump is growing bigger every day and becoming more noticeable. You might be getting stopped in the grocery store and seeing smiles from kind strangers. There is something so special about the way people slow down and acknowledge a pregnant belly. I really do feel that the sight of a pregnant mama grounds people in the beauty of humanity.

Although most loved ones and gawking strangers are well intended, sometimes the things that come out of people's mouths are straight up outrageous. "Twins!?" "You're huge!" "Are you sure you're eating enough for two?" "Prepare for exhaustion!" People can be so quick to spew their own misery on you. If you say you're having a home birth you may be bombarded with a home birth horror story or told about someone's traumatic birth. Sometimes the unwelcome commentary is not from

128

strangers we can walk away from, but from the people we love dearly whose approval and guidance we sincerely value.

Pregnancy is a time of profound softening in all senses of the word. Our body is preparing to open and our heart is expanding with love. This can come with greater sensitivity to other people's energy. I know personally I couldn't watch scary films while pregnant and I just wanted to be surrounded by positive and happy things. My capacity to filter out external negativity had changed, and I felt very protective of the state I was in.

No matter how confident you feel in your ability to create and maintain boundaries, parenthood will invite an opportunity to sharpen the skill every step of the way. I find that these situations arise as a gift from the universe to strengthen a crucial skill for parenthood. Children thrive when given space and freedom to explore physically and emotionally, knowing that a loving adult is maintaining the boundaries that keep them safe and feeling held. Part of being this container is modeling how we maintain our own personal boundaries. It is our work as parents to be that strong container for them, and if we don't have it for ourselves how can we create it for our children?

Bubble of Peace

This week I invite you to notice where in your life the need for stronger boundaries might be showing up for you. Perhaps you're feeling pressure to invite a certain family member into your birth space or to host guests after baby arrives. It is in great service to yourself, your pregnancy, and your baby to weed out the energy around you that is not serving you and to maintain a healthy boundary around your energy field.

ENERGETIC BOUNDARIES

This exercise can be done in conjunction with a longer meditation in a quiet space or be used in real time in social situations when it is needed most.

Take three deep breaths. With the first breath start to visualize an orb of light (whatever color you choose) expanding around you and with the next two inhales watch the orb engulf you completely with light and create a seal around you. You are now enclosed in your own amniotic sac just like your baby. It is strong and protective from the outside environment and engulfed in cleansing light. Place whatever energy, stories, or people that are not serving you outside of this energy field.

BIRTH BLESSINGS— A RITE OF PASSAGE

Women have gathered to celebrate rites of passage for centuries across almost every culture in different ways. Today in the United States, it's customary to celebrate the anticipated arrival of a baby by "showering" mom with baby gear. Baby showers today are inextricably linked to consumer culture and are reflective of the belief that gizmos and gadgets are what mothers need to feel prepared. These offerings to parents are rooted in love and the desire to help, but I can tell you with confidence that no number of items on a baby registry will ever come close to providing new parents what they really need in the early months of parenthood: support, connection, and nourishment.

Over the years I have seen mothers, myself included, choose to forgo the "traditional" baby shower and registry and instead invite their community to partake in a birth blessing ceremony that acknowledges the spiritual growth of the rite of passage at hand. Much like a wedding ceremony, a blessing circle unites the community and gives us a sense of purpose in supporting this family on the cusp of new beginnings. Birth is a spiritual transformation and true prenatal care is so much more than just doctor's visits and ultrasounds. Birth blessing gatherings have their roots in the Navajo traditional "Blessing Way" that imparts blessings of protection and connection through major life initiations.

When I was twenty weeks pregnant, my midwife and friends facilitated a ceremony for me that I will forever cherish. The day started with just an intimate group of a few of my closest girlfriends and my sisters. They blindfolded me, undressed me, and bathed me. As they lovingly cleansed my pregnant body they each voiced something they wished for me to wash away in my transition from maiden to mother: "fear of judgment," "control," "the need to please others," "worry." Next, they poured honey over me and surrounded me with blessings of the sweetness they hoped motherhood would bring. They then removed the blindfold and bathed me in a warm coconut milk wildflower bath. I was fed grapes off the vine and pampered like a goddess.

Later that day we gathered in a wider circle of friends and family. We sat in front of an altar where everyone brought objects from nature and a bead that they infused with a blessing. Everyone was sent home with a rose quartz birth blessing candle that they could light when they learned the news of Lou's arrival as a prayer for peaceful beginnings. The mother blessing not only centers the mother but also uplifts her support system, reminding them that they will be called on.

In the weeks that followed, I made a necklace out of the beads. As I strung each bead, I meditated on the qualities I saw in these women

132

that I hoped to embody as I stepped into motherhood. This necklace symbolized the circle and held the energy of all those whose love and support has carried me through. When labor began, I draped the beads around my neck and felt the strength of that sisterhood. The necklace now hangs above the bed where Lou sleeps and one day I will pass it on to her.

In a world of isolation that prides itself on individuality, being so intimately loved on can feel foreign and even vulnerable, but we are hungry for connection, for community, and to feel held by one another. Motherhood is a season of so much giving, to practice receiving is a valuable skill to help you fill up your cup.

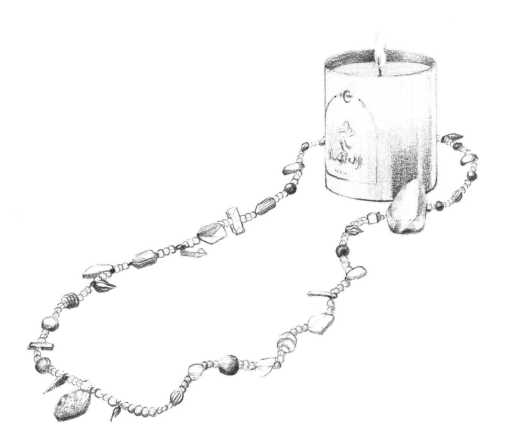

133

Creating Ritual & Ceremony

There are so many beautiful ways to create ritual and meaningful connection when honoring a pregnant mama. This week's activity is to bring together your village to create a meaningful ritual to prepare you for your rite of passage.

MANTRA PRAYER FLAGS

Give each guest a flag to engrave with words of encouragement. This can be hung in mama's birth space to remind her of the love she is surrounded by.

SHARE A POEM

Ask everyone to bring a poem to the circle that can be put into a scrapbook for mama to turn to for encouragement in pregnancy, birth, and motherhood.

CACAO CEREMONY

In many traditions, cacao is considered a sacred plant known for its "heart opening" medicine. Circle up with girlfriends, sing, laugh, dance, and set intentions while delighting over the richness of ceremonial cacao.

QUILTING

Each member of the circle gets a square piece of fabric to decorate, embroider, paint, or dye. The squares get sewn together as a quilt for mama to wrap herself in through pregnancy and birth and pass on to the baby.

COOKING

I once attended a baby shower where the host had printed several recipes from the postpartum cookbook *The First Forty Days* and put all the guests to work washing, chopping, and cooking nourishing stews for the expectant family. These meals were put into mason jars and stored in a deep freezer.

GESTATIONAL DIABETES SCREENING

Babies develop taste buds in the womb and studies show that what a mother eats in pregnancy can impact a baby's taste profile, so if you want your baby to eat his greens, now is the time to start leading by example and introducing your baby to an array of flavors.

Between twenty-four and twenty-eight weeks you will be screened for gestational diabetes (GD), which impacts around 14 percent of pregnancies. If left unmanaged, it is associated with increased risks for both mom and baby. Those who are overweight, have a family history of type 2 diabetes, or are over the age of thirty-five have a higher likelihood of testing positive for GD. However, nearly half of women diagnosed with GD don't fall into these categories.

GD is detected through a blood test taken after consuming a sugary drink (glucola), which spikes your blood sugar to see how your insulin levels respond. Unfortunately, this test often produces false negative and false positive results. Women who eat a low-glycemic diet are actually more likely to have a false positive because their body is not used to having to process such high levels of glucose so quickly. On top of that, the drink that is given to expecting mothers contains ingredients I would never want to consume in pregnancy (or at any other time, for that matter). If you read the label for this drink you will see brominated soybean oil, which is banned in the EU and Japan. Bromine inhibits thyroid function, irritates mucous membranes, and can cause neurological symptoms. It is colored with food dyes linked to cancer, hyperactivity, and allergic reactions. In recent years, alternative drinks with less additives have emerged that mothers can source online.

The metabolism changes in pregnancy to ensure the baby is getting the nutrients he needs. However, this becomes an issue when maternal diet and lifestyle do not support healthy blood sugar levels and mom experiences insulin resistance. The good news is that most people can successfully manage gestational diabetes without medication[59] and go on to have a healthy pregnancy by simply making changes to their diet and lifestyle.

Instead of going the conventional route and taking the glucose drink followed by a blood test, I opted to test my own levels at home with a blood sugar monitor with the support of my midwife. I tested my blood sugar in the morning immediately upon waking and an hour after each meal for a full week. This method allowed me to learn about how different foods impacted my blood sugar levels throughout the day. What I discovered was that my post-meal levels were in a healthy range, but my fasting glucose in the morning was higher than it should be. Having a hard-boiled egg at around 10 p.m. before going to bed was enough to sustain me through the night and wake up with optimal blood sugar levels.

When it comes to managing GD, the American Diabetes Association suggests expectant mothers with gestational diabetes eat 60 grams of carbohydrates at each meal. Since we know that carbohydrates turn into glucose in the body, which is not well tolerated for those with diabetes, why then would they recommend consuming even more glucose than the diagnostic drink itself?

Those who detect blood sugar levels out of range should prioritize meals with optimal protein and healthy fat intake and limit high-glycemic foods such as grains, anything made with flour, beans, potatoes, winter squash, sweet potatoes, and sugar. By monitoring your post-meal blood sugar you can get a better idea of how certain foods impact your levels and see for yourself how well-balanced meals can allow for more variety in your diet. Refer to Week 7 for more ideas for balanced meals and snacks.

In addition to nutrition, it is well studied that stress management and daily exercise can reduce the need for insulin. Commit to taking a brisk walk daily that gets your heart rate up. Supplementing with magnesium, probiotics, vitamin D, and cinnamon can also help stabilize blood sugar.

Hardy Pregnancy Salad

This salad Johnathan makes was one of my biggest pregnancy cravings. It is packed with protein and fat for healthy blood sugar balance and made me feel energized through every trimester.

2 or 3 large handfuls organic salad greens (arugula is my favorite)

4 slices pastured bacon, cooked and chopped

1 ripe avocado, peeled, pitted, and mashed

Toasted sesame seeds

Sauerkraut

2 stalks hearts of palm

½ cucumber, sliced or diced

2 hard-boiled eggs, sliced

Generous squeeze of fresh lemon

1½ tsp extra-virgin olive oil

Salt

Combine all the ingredients in a salad bowl and toss until thoroughly mixed.

A NOTE ABOUT BACON

I suggest oven-cooking pasture-raised bacon. This method makes the most of this delicious and nutritionally dense ingredient. Place the bacon slices on a parchment-lined baking sheet and bake at 400°F [200°C] for 15 to 20 minutes. Once the bacon is cooked, transfer it to a plate or cutting board. Position a small fine-mesh sieve over the mouth of a mason jar, and carefully pour the liquid gold cooking fat from the pan into the jar. This rendered fat can be stored in the fridge and used as a flavorful cooking fat for future culinary adventures.

139

Creating Balance Beyond Nutrition

Balancing blood sugar through balanced meals is just one of many tools at our disposal to improve our well-being, but oftentimes we also need to address imbalances in our personal life, work, or relationships to find harmony. I invite you to spend some time journaling about the areas of your life beyond nutrition that could benefit from more balance.

YOGA FOR PREGNANCY

You're nearly to the third trimester! For some the burst of energy that comes in the second trimester sticks around, while others start to feel pretty weighed down (literally!) as their growing baby gets bigger and bigger. As your organs and bones continue to shift, creating more space for your baby to grow, now is an excellent time to get in the habit of stretching and walking daily in preparation for birth. With a focus on gentle strengthening, flexibility, and breath, prenatal yoga is a wonderful tool to relieve tension and keep muscle aches and pains at bay. Here are some daily exercises to turn to.

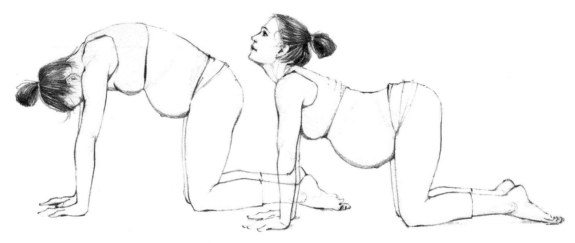

Cat-cow: This stretch can help improve spine mobility and core strength while reliving tension in the back.

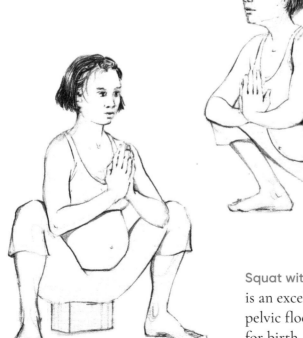

Squat with blocks: A supported squat is an excellent way to lengthen the pelvic floor muscles in preparation for birth.

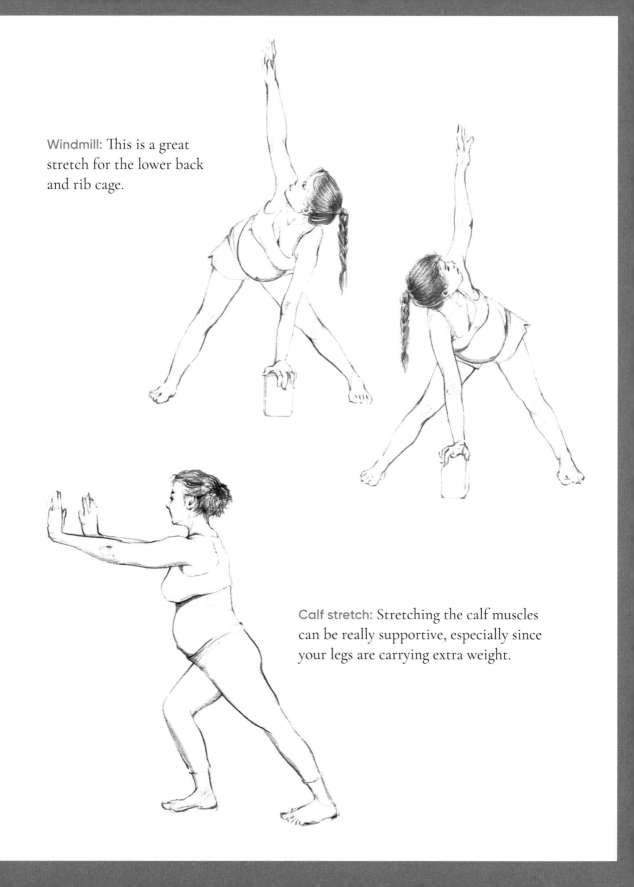

Windmill: This is a great stretch for the lower back and rib cage.

Calf stretch: Stretching the calf muscles can be really supportive, especially since your legs are carrying extra weight.

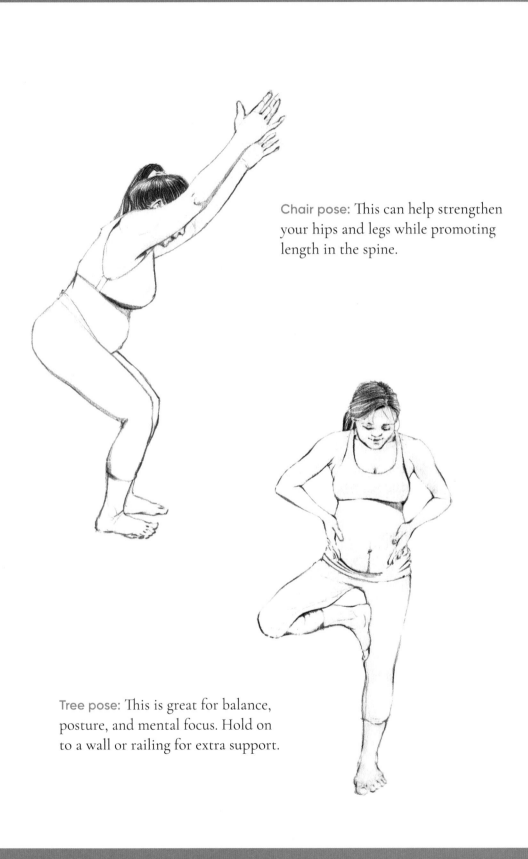

Chair pose: This can help strengthen your hips and legs while promoting length in the spine.

Tree pose: This is great for balance, posture, and mental focus. Hold on to a wall or railing for extra support.

RELAXIN

Relaxin is a hormone released by your placenta through pregnancy and birth to help loosen the ligaments that hold the pelvic bones together, facilitating expansion and allowing your body to accommodate the physical changes of growing a human. When it comes time for birth, this hormone promotes the softening of your cervix. You may find you are more flexible (or clumsy) in pregnancy because of the increase of this hormone. Utilize blocks when stretching to avoid hyperextension.

VITAMINS AND MINERALS TO CONSIDER IN PREPARATION FOR THE THIRD TRIMESTER

As your third trimester approaches here are some important nutrients to focus on for you and your baby's well-being. The food and supplements we consume in pregnancy help to build stores in our breast-milk that continue to nourish your little one even when they are on the other side.

Omega-3s: Omega-3s play an important role in baby's brain development and cognitive abilities, including language, memory, and attention. In fact, a baby's brain is made up of 60 percent fat, specifically DHA. Healthy fats also support mama's brain and help prevent postpartum depression. Optimal levels will also enrich your breast milk and decrease the risk of preeclampsia. Omega-3s are abundant in fish, with salmon roe being one of the greatest sources. There are valid concerns regarding mercury toxicity with excessive fish intake. However, the research shows that cognitive benefits of seafood consumption in pregnancy are high despite greater mercury exposure. • Where to find it: *Wild salmon, cooked oysters, cod, sardines*

145

Vitamin D3: On average, about 50 percent of women are deficient in vitamin D mostly because we are not getting nearly enough sunshine in our daily routines. Adequate vitamin D levels have been shown to cut the risk of preterm birth by half, protect against infection, promote proper placenta development and function, and reduce the risk of gestational diabetes and preeclampsia. Babies born with low vitamin D levels are shown to have an increased incidence of autoimmune disease, asthma, and poor language development. Every single food source of D3 contains fat and cholesterol, which makes sense because vitamin D is a fat-soluble vitamin. The app D Minder can help you decide on the most optimal time to be outside without sunscreen for you to receive the best absorption of the sun's healing rays. Consider getting your vitamin D levels tested throughout pregnancy so you can supplement appropriately. • Where to find it: *Sunshine, mackerel, wild salmon, cod liver oil*

Vitamin K2: Vitamin K2 works in tandem with calcium to help support bone formation and is also essential for proper blood clotting. Although modern breast milk is commonly deficient, when mama's vitamin K2 levels are optimal, high levels of K2 are transported to newborns via colostrum and breast milk. Because K2 helps deliver calcium where it needs to be in the body, it may help play a role in preventing calcium deposits in the placenta, which is often labeled as a sign of an "aging placenta," resulting in induction. • Where to find it: *Natto, beef liver, pork, chlorella, spirulina*

Annie's Beef Liver Pâté

This is a recipe from my friend Annie Whitehouse, who is an incredible Ayurvedic-trained postpartum doula and chef. Beef liver is a nutritional powerhouse and an excellent source of iron, choline, B12, folate, and selenium. My favorite way to enjoy it is by the spoonful, spreading it on fresh sourdough bread or seeded crackers. I also love mixing it into dishes for a boost of nutrients.

1 lb [455 g] pasture-raised grass-fed beef liver

1 Tbsp ghee, plus more as needed

Salt and pepper

3 cloves garlic, chopped

3 Tbsp chopped fresh herbs (thyme, rosemary, sage, or a mixture)

1 lb [455 g] unsalted grass-fed butter

Chop the liver into 2 in [5 cm] pieces, removing any tough membranes.

Melt the ghee in a pan over medium heat and add the liver. Season with salt and pepper. Sauté until almost cooked through, then add the chopped garlic and herbs. Cook until the liver is no longer pink in the middle. Let cool for a few minutes.

Transfer the liver mixture to a high-speed blender or food processor and blend, adding 1 Tbsp of butter at a time until completely smooth. This process can take up to 10 minutes. Your blender might need a break in between!

Taste and season with salt to your liking.

This will yield about four 8 oz mason jars.

Transfer to a glass containers and cover with a thin layer of melted ghee to keep your pâté fresh for up to a week in the fridge. It also freezes well.

RHESUS NEGATIVE (RH-)

By now you have probably received some bloodwork to determine whether or not your blood type is Rh-. If you have a positive blood type, this doesn't pertain to you, but if you have a negative blood type and your partner has a positive blood type, then you will be offered an injection of Anti-D in pregnancy and after birth to prevent your body from mounting an immune response if your Rh- blood comes in contact with the Rh+ blood of your baby. Incompatible blood mixing does not impact a current pregnancy but can lead to increased risk of complications in subsequent ones. Since you and your baby don't share a circulatory system, it is unlikely that any blood mixing will happen during pregnancy in the absence of abdominal injury or trauma. Due to the very minimal risk of blood mixing in pregnancy and valid concerns of a class C blood product that lacks safety studies in utero, many women choose to opt out of the shot in pregnancy but will choose to receive Anti-D after birth to protect future pregnancies in the event blood mixing has taken place at birth. It is wise to first determine your baby's blood type. If your baby is also Rh- there is no benefit to getting the injection. Either way, the choice is yours.

THE LOVE HORMONE

You know that feeling when you are deep in blissful love, perhaps laughing so hard with friends that tears come out of your eyes, receiving a long embrace from a loved one, stepping into a warm bath after a long day, or being greeted by your dog when you walk in the door. Those happy feelings all release a hormone in the body called oxytocin. You may know of oxytocin as the "love hormone" because it is also produced when making love. Midwives often say, "The same thing that makes the baby, brings the baby" because oxytocin plays a critical role in sex and in the birth process.

Oxytocin is the hormone that stimulates the uterine contractions necessary to birth your baby. During and immediately following childbirth a massive surge of oxytocin takes place. Looking deep into the eyes of your baby for the very first time sends this hormone surging and facilitates bonding, breast milk production, and the birth of your placenta. It also shrinks down the uterus to manage bleeding.

149

Although there are many hormones at play during birth, oxytocin deserves the spotlight because it is the proof that the environment you give birth in, the support you receive, and your feelings of safety directly contribute to the biological function of birth and the well-being of mama and baby. Oxytocin is the reason why being in an intimate space surrounded by trust and respect is crucial and why soothing music,[60] loving touch, and dim lighting do a lot more than generate nice photos and positive memories. An oxytocin ambience quite literally allows the innate brilliance of birth to unfold as intended.

The role of oxytocin also reminds us that an undisturbed mother-baby dyad after birth is essential. Skin-to-skin contact, eye gazing, and basking in each other's pheromones fires off oxytocin to complete the birth process and begin the breastfeeding journey. This is why my greatest birth advice is to simply follow the oxytocin. Over the next few weeks, I will walk you through the physiology of labor and all of your options so that you can set yourself up for a healthy and harmonious birth centering the hormone of love and connection.

Calling on Oxytocin

This week's activity is to engage in at least one oxytocin-inducing activity a day (sex, cardio, cuddles... the choice is yours). Get well acquainted with this feel-good love hormone that is here to support you through pregnancy, birth, and beyond.

Journal about what turns you on and how your understanding of the role of oxytocin in labor informs how you envision birthing.

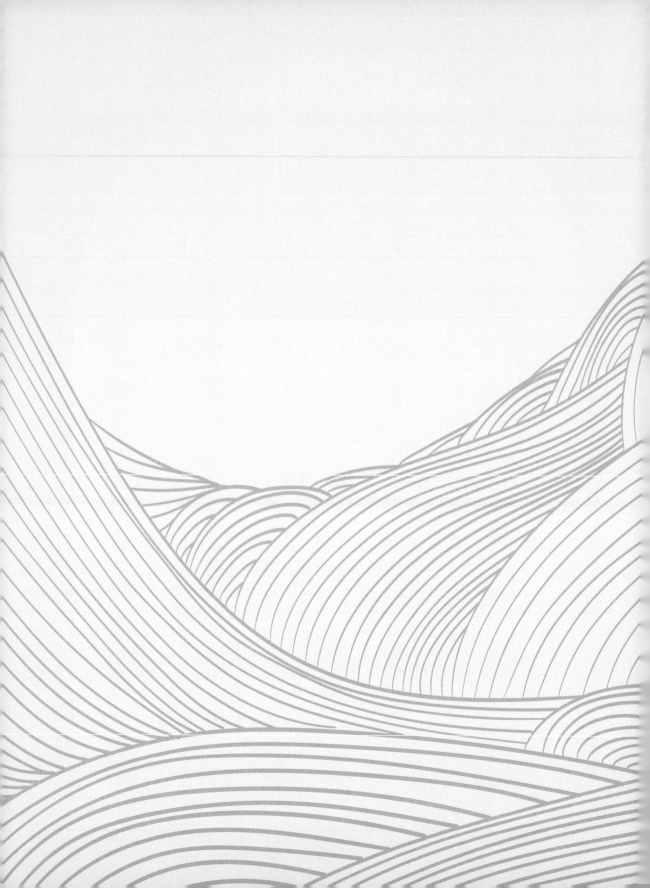

THIRD TRIMESTER

"Every midwife knows that not until a mother's womb softens from the pain of labor will a way unfold and the infant finds that opening to be born. Oh friend! There is treasure in your heart, it is heavy with child. Listen. All the awakened ones, like trusted midwives are saying, 'welcome this pain.' It opens the dark passage of Grace."

RUMI

LABOR'S UNFOLDING

EARLY LABOR

During labor, as the love hormone oxytocin surges through you, the uterus contracts, encouraging the cervix to soften, shorten, and open for baby's descent through the birth canal. Early labor can be long (hours or even days). For women who have given birth before, labor tends to be shorter, but of course this is not always the case for everyone.[61] Contractions may stop and start and have irregular patterns, usually lasting thirty to sixty seconds. Although early labor contractions can feel intense right from the start, they generally don't demand all of your attention and there is greater space for rest between them.

Women will often ask me how they can shorten the duration of labor and my answer is, don't start the clock. In early labor it is best to carry on with your usual routine. If labor begins at night, keep the lights down and rest as much as you can between each wave. You may

154

have a long road ahead and you will need all the energy you can get. Labor will demand the attention it needs, and if it isn't all-consuming it's probably still early labor.

When to Go to the Hospital

If you are planning a hospital birth and wondering how you will know when it is time to go to the hospital, this is a question only you can really answer. There comes a time in labor when you want to be in the place you plan to give birth in and that urge will guide you. If you want to avoid unnecessary intervention, it is in your best interest to labor in the comfort of your home for as long as possible. As a doula I observe the rhythm of labor, the cadence and intensity of contractions, and the mom's state. Most importantly I listen to the mother and trust that she knows when she is ready.

ACTIVE LABOR

Active labor builds in intensity, creating deeper sensations. These contractions generally last a full minute and you may notice a more consistent pattern. Vomiting, bloody show, and trembling can also be indications of active labor. As your focus turns inward, you will be less communicative but more audible with each contraction. Active labor changes your perception of time and brings you to an altered state of consciousness that allows you to drop out of your head and into your body. One cannot simply think their way through labor. When our minds get out of the way, the primal self takes hold and from there birth can unfold.

Dilation

A completely dilated cervix is considered 10 centimeters, but it is important to note that you don't have to know how dilated you are to give birth. Your cervical dilation can only be measured by an internal vaginal exam by a nurse, doctor, or midwife using their fingers to estimate the openness of your cervix. Cervical exams are uncomfortable and not always accurate. Although there are instances where this exam may be helpful in making decisions, it truthfully gives us very little information about the progress of labor. (Plus it can increase your risk of infection.) The textbooks will tell you that a laboring woman is to dilate 1 centimeter every one to two hours, but some dilate from 1 to 10 centimeters in a couple of hours and others in a couple of days. These unfounded expectations imposed on a process as nuanced as life itself can lead women down a cascade of interventions and leave them feeling defeated for not meeting these arbitrary benchmarks. When I was in labor I did not want anyone's fingers anywhere near my vagina and I knew that knowing how dilated I was would only be disruptive for me, so I chose to opt out altogether.

A Note on Timing Contractions

Active labor is generally determined by the 3-1-1 rule, meaning a contraction every three minutes, lasting a full minute, with the pattern staying consistent for a full hour. This pattern can sometimes be a reliable way of assessing progress; it can also be meaningless. Birth does not operate within a framework of the man-made constructs of time. There is no app, clock, or monitor more reliable than the inner wisdom of a mama. It will serve you well in labor to ditch the timer and instead note the rhythms at play.

TRANSITION

Transition is the final stage of active labor before the urge to push. This period is often accompanied by an overwhelming surge of emotion and intense physical sensation. Transition pushes you beyond the threshold of what you thought you were capable of. This is the space where you must gather all your strength and travel to another dimension to get your baby. As your body makes way for new life, there's an engulfing awareness that every aspect of yourself will be forever changed. Tears may flow and doubt may consume you, but this is all part of the process of the great surrender. You may feel like you are on the verge of death and that is because you are putting the maiden to rest to make way for the birth of a mother.

PUSHING

Pushing is a reflex; without an epidural your body will automatically know when and how to push. Much like projectile vomiting, the pushing reflex can't be stopped. For some the pushing stage is minutes long, and for others it can be hours. As the baby makes his way through the birth canal, his head stretches mom's perineum. This tight squeeze prepares his brain and lungs for the outside world.

The strong sensations of unmedicated labor will lead you to the optimal position in which to push and deliver your baby. You do not have to give birth on your back and if your doctor tells you that you do . . . get a new doctor! Below are some pushing positions that I see women gravitate to, but only you know the best position for you, so let your body and baby lead you to that place.

Pushing Positions

When pushing you should never feel confined to one position but rather be able to move through different positions to find where you feel most comfortable. Movement through labor and pushing will support baby's descent through the pelvis.

157

Runner's lunge: This maximizes space in the pelvis and is recommended in the event of a shoulder dystocia to free baby's shoulder.

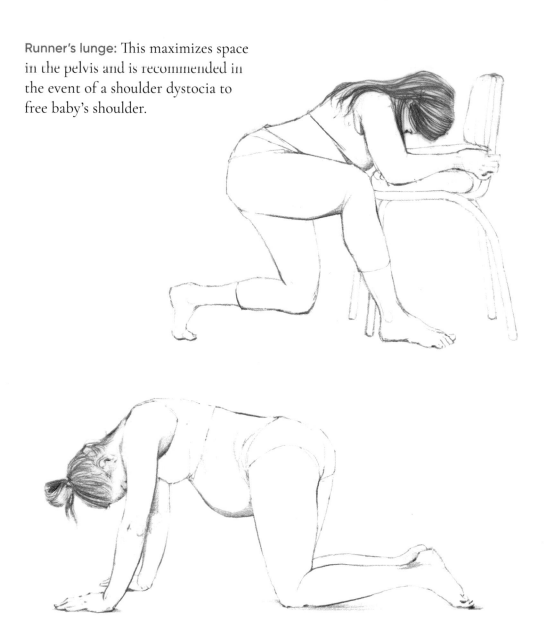

On all fours: This position keeps the hips nice and wide allowing the tailbone to ungulate back, making lots of space for baby.

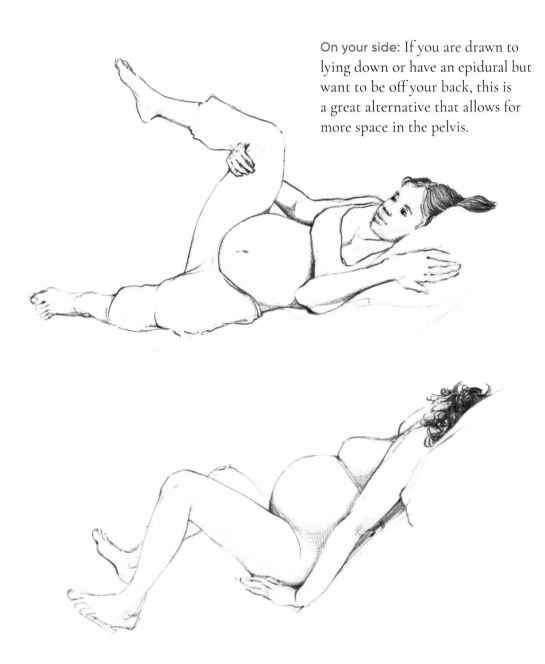

On your side: If you are drawn to lying down or have an epidural but want to be off your back, this is a great alternative that allows for more space in the pelvis.

Supine: Although this position tends to get a bad rap, it is actually a position that some women gravitate toward when birthing, and there is nothing wrong with birthing on your back as long as it is your preference and not for your provider's ease.

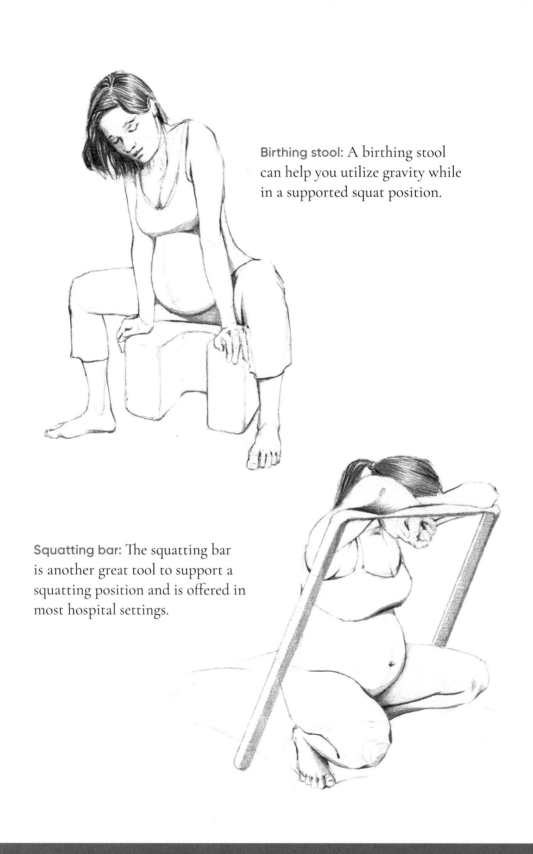

Birthing stool: A birthing stool can help you utilize gravity while in a supported squat position.

Squatting bar: The squatting bar is another great tool to support a squatting position and is offered in most hospital settings.

Toward the end of this process your baby's head will come under your pubic bone and begin to crown. With this sensation you may feel the impulse to stop pushing, as this allows your baby's head to emerge slowly to prevent tearing. Once his head is out, the next contraction will help rotate his shoulders so he can navigate through the pelvis and be born. This process is perfectly designed and for the most part does not require any hands-on assistance. Although common obstetrical practice is to "help" baby's shoulders rotate by manually guiding baby out, this may result in vaginal tearing and is unnecessary in the absence of a shoulder dystocia (which happens in less than 2 percent of deliveries). You can birth your baby slowly into your own loving hands or the hands of your partner in any position you like. Baby should be brought to your bare chest immediately with his cord kept intact. Refer to Week 17 for more information on cord cutting.

When Will My Waters Release?

You will have to wait and see! Your water can break before labor begins, at any point during labor, or it can remain intact with your baby born inside. This is called an en caul birth, a rare phenomenon that is considered auspicious in many cultures. You may experience the unmistakable "Hollywood gush" or just a small amount of fluid trickling down your leg. All scenarios are healthy variations of normal.

Only about 15 percent of women have their water break before the onset of labor and 90 percent of those women will go into labor naturally within forty-eight hours.[62] The current guidelines within the obstetrical model are to induce labor immediately after the water breaks to prevent infection now that the protective amniotic environment is no longer sealed off. (For this reason, it is in your best interest not to allow a clinician to break your bag of waters.) Studies show that after twenty-four hours, risk of infection may increase and therefore active management is recommended. However, the studies that inform this recommendation leave out a crucial confounding factor: there is a 250 percent increase in neonatal infection with vaginal exams at trial entry.[63] More recent studies have indicated that waiting for up to two or three days for labor to begin on its own is also an evidence-based option if mom and baby are doing well and meet certain criteria. Since there is no risk-free option, it is important that each mother consider her own preferences and individual circumstances to make an informed decision. Regardless of the path you choose, remember that the most effective way to prevent infection after your water breaks is to avoid cervical exams.

When your water breaks, you will want to look at the color of the fluid. Brown or green fluid indicates the presence of meconium, baby's first poop. Meconium is passed prior to delivery in 15 to 40 percent of pregnancies depending on gestational age. Often meconium-stained fluid is not indicative of a problem and reflects the fully developed and working digestive system of your baby. In a small number of cases meconium may signal fetal distress, so be sure to keep your provider informed. The main concern is the inhalation of meconium upon birth interfering with respiration, and this is a rare occurrence called meconium aspiration syndrome (MAS). Premature babies are at greater risk and the risk is higher when breathing is constricted, causing the baby to gasp and inhale the meconium at birth. When meconium is present it is all the more reason to create a relaxing birth environment, keep the cord intact, and avoid interventions that are associated with fetal distress, such as induction and immediate cord clamping.

PLACENTA BIRTH

This stage of labor happens after your baby is born. Hormones signal to the placenta to detach from the uterine wall, and the surge of oxytocin that takes place when you are skin-to-skin with your baby stimulates contractions to support the birth of the placenta. These contractions are far less intense than labor contractions but are generally felt more with each subsequent pregnancy. Delivering the placenta may require a small push but often comes out without much effort. For some the placenta is born shortly after the baby and for others it can take an hour or even longer. Care providers in hospital settings don't have much experience patiently allowing the placenta birth, so therefore active management tends to be the default.

An actively managed placenta birth includes IV administration of Pitocin and cord traction, where the provider pulls the placenta out by tugging at the cord. If the placenta has not yet detached this can put the mother at greater risk of hemorrhage or cause damage to the uterus. You can request to birth your placenta on your own time in whatever position you choose. Perhaps you want to guide your own placenta out when it's ready.

POOPING IN LABOR

If you have been worried about the prospect of pooping in labor, you're not alone. If you are just learning that this is a thing, sorry to be the one to bring you up to speed. The good news is there's nothing to worry about. As your baby descends into the birth canal he pushes onto your bowels, and together with your pushing efforts this can lead to a bowel movement. Pooping while you push is indicative of good progress! Nearly everyone does it and frankly you probably won't ever know you did. To be honest, a baby's exposure to mom's fecal matter at birth may even be beneficial to the development of their microbiome.

Get Comfortable Not Having All the Answers

Sitting with the uncertainty of when and how your birth will unfold is uncomfortable in a world of instant gratification fixated on answers. Babies carry their own wisdom, and this process is just as much theirs as it is yours.

This week I want you to reflect on any assumptions or expectations you are holding on to about birth. Ask yourself where and how in your life you can practice letting go of the expectation that things will happen within a certain time frame or look a certain way. How can you practice getting more comfortable with not having all the answers? Think back to a time in your life where you didn't have the answers, a time where you were invited to surrender to the unknown. What did that bring up within you, and how did you navigate the discomfort? If you could go back in time knowing what you know now, what would you tell that version of yourself?

YOUR BIRTH INTENTIONS

Over the next two weeks I will walk you through creating your birth plan or what I like to call Birth Intentions. Whether you are birthing at home or at a hospital, you have many options available to you and choices to make. Being well informed about the birth process and your rights will prepare you to advocate for yourself and will help set you up for an empowered birth on your terms. Remember, you are the authority when it comes to your body and your baby. Your provider should always acknowledge that you have the legal right to consent.

The birth process is as magnificently unique as each individual being. This is why I prefer the term Birth Intentions. That said, you absolutely can prioritize a healthy and positive birth experience and set yourself up to be supported by those who will honor your needs and treat you with dignity. Where you choose to birth, who is present, and how you utilize interventions all have an impact on how your birth unfolds. Here are some reasons why I recommend creating your Birth Intentions.

When you thoughtfully familiarize yourself with the different interventions, medications, and procedures available, you can consider how these options may pose risks or provide benefits to you and your baby. Labor is all-consuming and you don't want to be gathering this information on the spot or in the event of an unexpected hospital transfer.

If you are giving birth at home, it is equally important to have a dialogue with your midwife about how you expect her to show up in your birth space and what your preferences are. Not all midwives have the same approach to birth.

Creating Birth Intentions that clearly outline what is important to you is arguably more useful prior to labor. You can bring this sheet to your doctor or midwife during one of your prenatal visits as a tool for assessing how your provider approaches birth and whether you are the right fit for one another. For example, if your Birth Intentions say you would like to birth in any position but your doctor says that that is "not allowed," you can make the switch to a provider who (a) understands that they should follow your lead regarding the position you want to birth in and (b) has the necessary skills to catch your baby in any position you please.

SOVEREIGN BIRTH

Although informed consent is a fundamental legal right that should not have to come with a caveat, I want to be real with you. Hospitals have guidelines that they expect their patients to follow and licensed doctors and midwives must abide by the rules of the medical board or risk losing their license. This means that women don't always have full autonomy when birthing within the system. No one can force you to do anything you don't want to do, but they can deny you care if your wishes don't align with policy.

For example, some hospitals don't support vaginal birth after Cesarean or breech delivery, in California midwives must pass off their clients to an OB past forty-two weeks of pregnancy, and in New York Child Protective Services will be called if you attempt to opt out of prophylactic administration of newborn antibiotics because the treatment is required by law. You see, informed consent does not really exist unconditionally. This is why more and more women are turning to home birth and free birth.

One of the many reasons why I chose to give birth at home with an autonomous midwife was to have complete sovereignty over my body and baby. I did not want to have to unnecessarily expend any energy defending my legal rights while I was in labor, as I knew this would disrupt the healthy physiological process of my birth. With that said, home birth or free birth is not for everyone, and I have been a part of many empowered hospital births where parents have been respected in their choices by successfully advocating for themselves and had the birth of their dreams. It all begins with how you prepare and whom you choose to support you.

Let's walk through some of the options available to you and the tools to navigate your choices no matter where you decide to give birth.

WHAT TO INCLUDE IN YOUR BIRTH INTENTIONS

General information: At the top of the Birth Intentions document, I advise my clients to include: name of their partner, support team, pediatrician's name, current supplement and medications, allergies, previous surgeries, and medical history. I also encourage a brief "about me" section. This can be a sentence or two about your pregnancy and anything you would like the hospital staff to know about you, assuming you'll arrive in active labor and won't be very chatty. In this section you may also want to thank your nurse for being a valuable part of your birth team. Approaching hospital staff with the spirit of collaboration goes a long way.

Your Birth Intentions are a moving and changing road map that moves and changes in accordance with your needs in the moment. Your partner should familiarize himself with your Birth Intentions so he can help you advocate for yourself in real time and understand why these choices are important to you.

Comfort measures: Week thirty-one we will be talking all about your options for pain management. Once you have a better idea of your pain management preferences, you can add them in here. Remember, nothing is set in stone. Keep in mind that 70 percent of women who give birth in the hospital utilize an epidural and it is a nurse's job to offer you pain medication. If you are wanting to avoid narcotics in labor or trying to delay the use, you may want to write something like: *Please don't offer pain medication to me; when/if I choose to utilize pain medication I will ask for it.* This reminds your support team that you and only you know when and if you need medical pain relief. When choosing your place of birth and provider you will want to make sure you have access to a birthing tub, shower, and freedom of movement at all times, which will allow for more comfort in labor.

Fetal monitoring and exams: Over the last few decades, women have become accustomed to continuous electronic fetal monitoring (EFM) during birth as part of the normal birth process. When giving birth in a hospital, the expectation is for all laboring women to be strapped to a continuous fetal monitor that is tethered to a computer monitor for the entire duration of labor. This allows nurses to monitor from another room because the baby's heartbeat is projected onto the monitor, providing convenience for a busy nurse. The ongoing record of vitals is also preferable for the hospital in the event of a malpractice lawsuit.

Being strapped to a monitor while in labor hinders your freedom of movement, which is essential for coping with pain and encouraging optimal fetal positioning. If you plan to give birth without pain medication, continuous fetal monitoring makes it very challenging to do so. Additionally, research shows that not all patients actually benefit from continuous fetal monitoring.[64] In low-risk pregnancies, continuously monitoring the baby is associated with an increase in Cesarean surgery and an increase in use of pain medications and does not improve rates of stillbirth, brain damage, NICU admission, or neurological injury. Opting out altogether will not be an option in a hospital setting, but you can request intermittent fetal monitoring with a handheld doppler. Have a conversation with your provider prior to labor to gauge their comfort level and whether the nursing staff will have access to a handheld doppler. A nurse cannot approve this request without the go-ahead from your doctor. A handheld doppler, unlike an EFM strap, allows you to move around as desired as the nurse collects fetal tones for charting.

BYOG: BRING YOUR OWN GOWN

If you're giving birth in a hospital you will be in the only unit in that hospital that is not dedicated to treating illness and emergencies. The labor and delivery unit is the only part of the hospital full of healthy people celebrating the best day of their life! Hospital gowns are symbolic of sickness and have no place at your birth. You are walking into your most powerful day, so dress for the occasion! Pack your own comfortable clothing to wear during labor and delivery. They make labor gowns that accommodate epidural placement, easy skin-to-skin contact, breastfeeding, and baby monitoring without the clinical

169

feeling. You can also opt for a robe, button-down shirt, sports bra, or just your birthday suit. Don't forget cozy socks or slippers.

EATING IN LABOR

Studies show that when given the option, 95 percent of women choose to eat in labor. However, in the United States, 60 percent of women without an epidural and 83 percent with an epidural are limited to just ice chips and clear fluids.

Proper nourishment in labor can help strengthen contractions (the uterus is mostly made of muscle tissue) and prevent exhaustion. Evidence has shown that unrestricted eating in labor results in shorter labors and higher maternal satisfaction, while restricting food can cause greater pain and stress. Why, then, are so many told they shouldn't eat in labor? This policy is based on practices from the 1940s where women were often unconscious or put under "twilight sleep" to birth. The risk of aspiration was also higher due to the lack of sophistication of anesthetics and available surgical tools we have today.

Some have no desire to eat in labor while others crave nutrients to keep them energized. In early labor I recommend easy-to-digest foods rich in protein and healthy fats to keep your blood sugar stable. In active labor, it is best to turn to healthful natural sugars such as fruit, raw honey, applesauce, and coconut. As always, listening to your body is most important!

IN THE CASE OF A CESAREAN

In pregnancy or during labor certain situations may arise where Cesarean birth becomes the best route of delivery for the well-being of mom and baby. Cesarean birth can undoubtedly be a lifesaving procedure when used appropriately. The World Health Organization states that a national Cesarean rate that reflects proper use is between

10 and 15 percent. Yet today in the United States it is at 30 percent and in some states as high as 50 percent.[65] The Cesarean delivery rate has increased 500 percent since 1970! This is reflective of a system where a woman is at a significantly higher risk of Cesarean delivery than proven medically necessary. It is widely abused and overutilized in the United States, resulting in an increase in complications and risks for mothers and babies.

Cesarean section is a major abdominal surgery that results in a longer hospital stay and a more challenging recovery. The operation is associated with greater blood loss, risk of hemorrhage, infection, and blood clots, and the maternal death rate after a Cesarean delivery is three to four times higher than a vaginal delivery. A mother who gives birth via Cesarean is also more likely to experience ectopic pregnancy, placenta previa, placenta accreta, placental abruption, emergency hysterectomy, and uterine rupture in subsequent pregnancies. Babies born via Cesarean tend to have more difficulty breathing upon birth and face greater challenges breastfeeding. The maternal vaginal microbiota provides newborns with a greater variety of colonizing microorganisms responsible for boosting and preparing the immune system,[66] which is why it is believed that babies born via Cesarean are at greater risk of developing asthma, diabetes, and allergies.[67]

The medicalization of birth is one of the primary factors for the rising Cesarean rate. OB-GYNs are skilled surgeons, but not all are experts in the healthy, natural birth process, which is why we see lower Cesarean rates under the midwifery care model. Common labor interventions such as induction and epidural increase risks of complications that may lead to a Cesarean and restrict the physiological birth process. Additionally, hospitals get paid more for a Cesarean birth than a vaginal birth and are less likely to face litigation. It holds up better in court for a doctor to have performed a Cesarean regardless of the

171

outcome to demonstrate that they did everything possible to protect the mother and baby. There are many ways to reduce your chances of a Cesarean (by choosing the right care provider, hiring a doula, avoiding unnecessary intervention, giving birth at home, and moving around freely, to name a few).

No matter what route your baby takes to be born, it is always a sacred event that requires a great deal of strength from mothers. If a Cesarean birth becomes the best option for you or your baby, here are some preferences to consider for your Birth Intentions:

1	To remain as conscious as possible during delivery, please discuss anesthesia options with me.
2	I would like the drape to be lowered to see the birth.
3	I would like to do skin-to-skin contact in the OR and stay with my baby at all times.
4	I would like to play my own music.
5	I ask for the room to be quiet and to please avoid any small talk.
6	I ask for delayed cord clamping if possible.

Create Your Birth Intentions

Take all that you've learned so far and start to map out your own Birth Intentions document. Continue to gather information internally and externally. Discuss these choices with your partner.

BIRTH INTENTIONS CONTINUED: EXAMS AND PROCEDURES FOR BABY

After you give birth, the hospital staff will want to weigh, measure, and assess your baby. Immediate assessments of your baby's vitals can be observed while the baby is on your chest, and none of the exams and procedures beyond that should come between skin-to-skin bonding and breastfeeding. Request as much time as possible before your baby is taken off your chest for any routine exam. You may be excited to find

174

out how much your baby weighs, but that can and should wait! Skin-to-skin contact with mama is priority over anything else.

The following medications are administered as a blanket approach to all newborns born in the hospital regardless of risk factors present. As a parent, it is important to understand the benefits and risks as they apply to your individual circumstance before consenting to any routine procedure.

VITAMIN K

Babies are born with low levels of vitamin K and it is not understood why. In newborns with a hemorrhagic disease, low levels of vitamin K can result in life-threatening bleeding. To help prevent this, all newborns are given a vitamin K shot upon delivery. This intervention improves outcomes for the small percentage of babies with blood-clotting disorders. Some parents administer vitamin K orally without the preservatives that are present in the shot or opt out altogether given the limited data on any risks associated in giving a healthy newborn vitamin K at birth.

ANTIBIOTIC EYE OINTMENT

Erythromycin antibiotics are routinely put in newborns' eyes after birth to prevent blindness from exposure to chlamydia or gonorrhea in the birth canal. Sexually transmitted infections can be easily screened for in pregnancy, so it is therefore reasonable to decline this if in a monogamous relationship. A mother's healthy vaginal biome is not inherently dangerous to her baby and the risks of exposure to antibiotics unnecessarily outweigh any benefits.

175

HEPATITIS B VACCINE

Although over 99 percent of pregnant women test negative for hepatitis B, it is routine to be tested in pregnancy to prevent transmission at birth. Even though hepatitis B can be screened for in pregnancy, all babies are recommended the hepatitis B vaccine on the first day of life, which to me seems superfluous. Hepatitis B can only be spread through exchange of bodily fluids. If you and your partner test negative for hepatitis B and are not in a high-risk category, the risk of exposure to your newborns is negligible. According to the CDC, common side effects of the hepatitis B vaccine are fever, soreness, redness, or swelling at the injection site.[68] Whether or not these side effects interrupt early breastfeeding has not been studied, but I would assume so. More and more parents are choosing to delay or opt out of this vaccine altogether and questioning the necessity of a newborn receiving a vaccine to protect against a sexually transmitted infection.

Unfortunately, when it comes to vaccinations, parents don't feel they are able to discuss their concerns candidly with their pediatricians. State laws vary when it comes to informed consent around vaccinations, and providers are financially incentivized to persuade parents to go along with the CDC schedule. What was once a twelve-shot schedule in 1986 from birth to age eighteen is now a seventy-shot schedule. This change took place when vaccine manufacturers became indemnified against damages in the late 1980s. The long-term implications of the sixfold increase have not been studied.

NATURE'S VARNISH

You may have seen photos of freshly born babies covered in a white cream cheese–looking substance called vernix. Vernix is the Latin word for "varnish," which is essentially what it is. Some babies are born with a lot of it while others come out without any visible vernix on their skin. Babies who are born earlier tend to be born with more vernix. It protects your baby's skin from infection, helps regulate temperature, is high in antioxidant properties, and contains the familiar scent of the womb. It is beneficial to allow nature's varnish to remain on the baby for at least twenty-four hours after birth and refuse a baby bath in the hospital. Some mothers, myself included, choose to delay the first bath for a couple of weeks and to avoid use of any soaps in the early weeks of life.

JUST SAY NO TO BABY HATS

Hospital rooms can be chilly, and babies like to be warm and cozy. To help keep your baby warm nurses will put on a baby hat immediately upon arrival. This happens fast. So fast that it's almost as if the baby is born with a hat on. Being the pesky doula that I am, I quickly and gently remove the hat from baby's head and whisper into mama's ear, "Soak in those oxytocin-inducing pheromones on the top of your baby's beautiful head." When mama basks in the scents emitted from the top of her baby's head and feels her lips kiss the baby's soft skin underneath her chin, her body vibrates with love, and it is love that promotes oxytocin to help birth the placenta and shrink down the uterus. Skin-to-skin contact should be head to toe for the baby. Request the room be warmed and throw a warm blanket over the both of you to keep cozy.

Share Your Intentions

Continue to build on your Birth Intentions with all you've learned this week. Bring your Birth Intentions to your next visit with your doctor or midwife as a tool to prompt conversations that will give you more clarity on your provider's approach to birth. It is also important to share and discuss your preferences with your doula and partner. In the coming weeks we will cover additional topics that will continue to shape your Birth Intentions.

BIRTH IS NOT JUST A PHYSICAL EVENT

When Lily hired me she was eight months pregnant and planning a home birth with a midwife. After a few sessions together it became clear to me that her husband was going through a difficult time and was not showing up for their relationship. He missed our meetings, and I could tell she was feeling let down by him. She confided in me that she suspected he was using drugs again.

The evening Lily went into labor her husband was not home. When I arrived, I could tell that she was well into active labor, so I called her midwife and asked her to head over. Lily requested a vaginal exam; she was 9 centimeters dilated and in transition! If you remember from

179

the week on labor stages, 9 centimeters is close to the finish line. The medical textbooks would tell you that the last 1 centimeter of dilation "should" take place within the hour and the urge to push will follow immediately after. Between contractions she asked me to call her husband so that he knew the baby could be born any minute and to get home soon. He assured me over the phone that he would be on his way. Hours passed and her husband never showed up. Meanwhile, Lily's contractions came to a halt and no future "progress" was made for over six hours.

The midwife recognized that the stall in her labor was not a failure of her body nor an indication of a physical problem. Lily was face to face with her biggest tiger. She was being confronted with tremendous heartbreak and abandonment. Her external environment was impacting her labor. How could it not? After several more hours and unanswered phone calls came and went, the reality set in that he would not be coming. The wise midwife pulled me out of the room and said to me, "Let's give her some space. To bring her baby earthside she needs to know that she can do this alone." This midwife intuited exactly what Lily needed and within the next hour she felt the urge to push!

Lily went on to have a beautiful birth at home. There was no failure to progress. In fact, she succeeded in confronting spiritual and emotional adversity and faced her tiger. She needed that extra time to gather an even deeper level of strength before welcoming her baby girl. Had we been in the hospital, Lily would have been given Pitocin to help push labor along or perhaps a Cesarean. The most common reason for Cesareans is "failure to progress," but research has shown that over 50 percent of Cesarians that take place for this reason do not actually meet the criteria. Whether "failure to progress" should even be diagnosed at all is up for debate.

FAILURE TO BE PATIENT

The rate of induction of labor in the United States has risen from 9.6 percent in 1990 to 31 percent in 2020, and a large proportion of medically induced labors are for nonmedical reasons. This is a clear indication of a systemic failure to be patient. The assumption that all babies must be born by a designated date is as problematic as the assumption that every child must take their first step, say their first word, or learn to read at the same time. Most women are unsure of their conception date and therefore can't have complete certainty of a "due date," and a child's development is not in lockstep with imposed timelines or fear of liability.

It is understood that the start of labor is initiated by the baby, who releases a protein signaling to his mother his lungs' maturation. When labor begins on its own, it allows women to labor with optimal levels of endorphins and oxytocin release that increases the likelihood that labor and birth will progress successfully and that breastfeeding and attachment will get off to the best possible start.

Inductions also take place after the onset of labor if labor is not progressing in accordance with the provider's expectations and the obsolete timelines established in the 1950s by Dr. Emanuel Friedman. The study he conducted that set the standards used to assess labor progress included 500 women, 96 percent of whom were sedated with drugs and more than half the babies were delivered by forceps. This study did not look at physiological birth patterns but instead meddled with the birth process through intervention and unethical practices, such as vaginal exam while sedated. New guidelines and a return to common sense advocates for the abandonment of the term "failure to progress" and the understanding that labor length in and of itself is not indicative of a problem.

PITOCIN PITFALL

The most common method of induction is Pitocin, synthetic oxytocin, which is injected into the bloodstream via a continuous IV drip. Augmented labor looks and feels very different than natural labor. Although clinicians attempt to mimic the gradual increase of oxytocin by starting "low and slow," the medication utilized does not travel through the brain the way the natural oxytocin release does. This circumvents the endorphin release, creating far more intense contractions without the help of your body's innate "morphine-like effect." For this reason, induction usually goes hand in hand with the use of an epidural.

Many people don't realize that oxytocin is a drug commonly associated with preventable adverse perinatal outcomes. In 2007 it was added to the Institute for Safe Medication Practices' list of medications "bearing a heightened risk of harm." Stronger and more frequent contractions that are artificially produced can place undue strain on the baby, increasing the risks of hypoxia (low oxygen). For this reason, administration of synthetic oxytocin in labor always requires monitoring of the baby's heart rate to check for indications of fetal distress. Receiving synthetic oxytocin in labor may also increase the chance of postpartum hemorrhage. If induction takes place when a mother's cervix is not in a favorable condition for labor to begin, it can increase the likelihood of complications and cascading interventions.

INDUCING FOR A BIG BABY

With the increased use of ultrasound has come the greater speculation of a big baby. A baby is considered big when over 8 pounds 13 ounces [4 kg] and for providers, the fear of a big baby comes with the fear of shoulder dystocia, where the shoulders get stuck after the birth of the head. Care providers are apprehensive of dystocia because when it is poorly managed babies can lose oxygen or experience nerve injury. This injury is the most common reason for litigation in obstetrics.

It is important to understand that ultrasound has a margin of error and the assessment of a big baby will only be right half the time. Ultrasound weight calculations at the end of pregnancy may fall 15 percent above or below the actual weight.[69] Even if the speculation of a big baby is correct, this is not a problem considering the expansion and mobility of mom's pelvis that takes place in a labor when she is able to utilize movement and her innate ability to birth a big baby. "If a care provider thinks that you are going to have a big baby, this thought is sometimes more harmful than the actual big baby itself," states Rebecca Dekker of Evidence Based Birth. "This is because the suspicion of a big baby leads many care providers to manage labor in a way that increases the risk of Cesarean and complications."[70]

Although shoulder dystocia is more common with big babies, it can occur regardless of size and is impossible to predict. Birth via Cesarean for all babies would be the only way to remove the risk of dystocia altogether, but then the risks of additional complications present themselves. This brings us to the complex reality that in birth there are no risk-free options, which is why providers and parents should be well informed and prepared to manage shoulder dystocia if it presents itself regardless of size.

Over the past decade I have had the privilege of supporting my dear friend Kashia through the births of all three of her sons, Ezra (9 pounds [4.08 kg]), Otis (11 pounds [5 kg]), and Arlo (11.6 pounds [5.26 kg]). All her births took place in the hospital, unmedicated, vaginally, and under midwifery care. With each pregnancy the pressure to induce early or opt for a Cesarean increased, but she held firm in her inner knowing. "I give birth to big babies," she says. "At every birth

I've been lucky enough to have a nurse who truly believes in me and it's that encouragement that reminds me what I am capable of."

As I write this chapter, my phone dings. It's a mom from my Growing Together Circle sending a picture of her precious newborn baby, Nico. She writes, "I had a magical unmedicated hospital birth. Thank you for inspiring me. It was an absolute dream. Nico is 9 pounds 5 ounces [4.23 kg] and I had no idea because I hadn't had a scan since twenty weeks. I pushed him out in ten minutes with no tearing. It was the most healing experience of my life. I'm 5-foot-1 [1.55 m] with small hips, and my body knew exactly what to do."

THE ARRIVE TRIAL

In August of 2018 the ARRIVE Trial was published in the *New England Journal of Medicine*, stating that being induced at thirty-nine weeks lowers the risk of Cesarean by 4 percent, compared with waiting until at least forty weeks and five days to be induced. The comprehensive study seems to justify the superseding of Mother Nature's wisdom to prevent major abdominal surgery. As a result, this comprehensive review has shifted practices nationwide.

There are a few things worth taking into account regarding the ARRIVE Trial. Of the 22,533 participants eligible to participate, 27 percent (6,106) opted to be in the study. These mothers consented to having elective induction and were all planning medicalized births with epidurals. The study did not look at the correlation between those who were planning to birth naturally with those who were induced. The trial also failed to examine the difference between those who were induced and those who went into labor naturally. Most participants were either induced during the thirty-ninth week of pregnancy or at forty weeks and five days if they did not go into labor by then.

What is often left out of the discussion is that there are so many other ways to minimize your likelihood of having a Cesarean that are far more effective and less invasive. These evidence-based approaches include birthing out of hospital, having a doula, having a midwife, birthing in water, opting out of continuous fetal monitoring, and walking around during labor. The question we must ask is why aren't OBs advocating for the use of these techniques to reduce the likelihood of Cesarean like they are for early induction?

Conquer Limiting Beliefs

We have all been exposed to limiting beliefs around birth, whether from our own doctors, mothers, or the media. In my birth story I share how my first gynecologist visit at sixteen years old left me questioning my own ability to birth.

This week I invite you to get to the source of some of these limiting beliefs. Identify where these messages are coming from so you can discern what is your inner wisdom and what has been projected onto you. What stories are you holding on to about your body, your ability to birth, and your ability to mother in the way that is most authentic to you? Write down all the limiting beliefs you have or have been told onto a single piece of paper. Now turn the page and rewrite the belief to make it an affirmation. Write each one three times. Don't forget to rip up or burn the first page and keep the positive affirmations handy to revisit when needed.

EXAMPLE

Limiting belief
I am too small to birth my big baby vaginally.

Affirmation
MY BODY GROWS TO ACCOMMODATE
MY GROWING BABY SO I CAN BIRTH
HIM WITH EASE.

THE SENSATIONS OF LABOR

So many of us have been told time and time again how "painful" childbirth is. When we feel pain, it is usually a signal from the body that we are in danger or unwell. However, birth is really one of the only times where one feels such physical intensity under joyous and healthy circumstances. For this reason, I find it useful to detach from the word *pain* and its negative connotation when speaking about birth. I say this not to minimize its magnitude, but to help us reframe how we perceive it. I will be the first to tell you that even after years of attending births, I had greatly underestimated the physical sensation of birth, and when it came time for me to cross the threshold to motherhood I was deeply humbled. I begged for mercy and held on for dear life as labor dragged me through the depths of a realm I had never traveled to before, and in retrospect I wouldn't have changed a single thing about it.

Birth is a physical and emotional expansion. As you become a portal for the life of another being, you too are reborn. It is my belief that the

187

energy it takes to give life serves a purpose to help us access a boundless strength necessary for parenthood. It matches the magnitude of the transformation at hand. It's big work because it's BIG WORK!

ENDORPHINS AND OXYTOCIN WORKING TOGETHER

You may be familiar with endorphins as the feel-good hormone released during physical exercise. Endorphins are your body's natural pain reliever that activates the opioid receptors in the brain and helps reduce stress. Every runner knows that the runner's "high" isn't felt right away but usually kicks in after a few miles. The same happens in labor. The contractions stimulated by oxytocin bring on intense sensations that elicit the support of endorphins. This provides relief and has a feel-good effect that initiates more oxytocin, which helps labor progress further.

COMFORT MEASURES

In this chapter, I will share with you the different tools that can be utilized for relief in labor. Ultimately, what I have found to be the best approach to support a laboring woman is simply not disturbing her. Your body will innately writhe in response to labor to help facilitate birth. Following your body's lead with the freedom to move as you please in a peaceful and private environment is paramount.

Ask your birth team to support you in creating a sanctuary of trust and encouragement and to follow your lead. Dimming the lights, burning candles, and playing calming music will help you drop into the zone. Ask yourself what you need to feel safe so that you can drop in and ride the waves of labor.

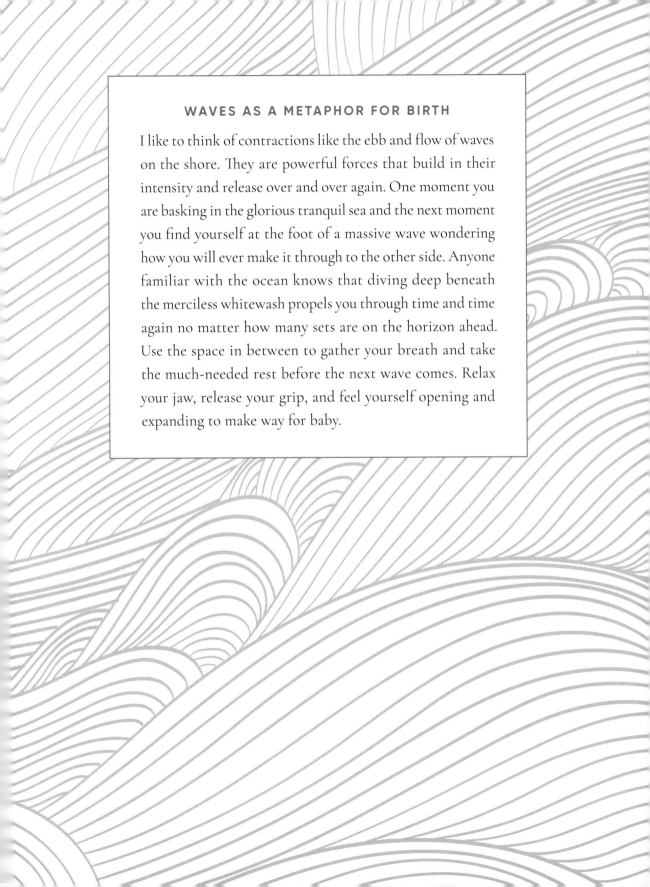

WAVES AS A METAPHOR FOR BIRTH

I like to think of contractions like the ebb and flow of waves on the shore. They are powerful forces that build in their intensity and release over and over again. One moment you are basking in the glorious tranquil sea and the next moment you find yourself at the foot of a massive wave wondering how you will ever make it through to the other side. Anyone familiar with the ocean knows that diving deep beneath the merciless whitewash propels you through time and time again no matter how many sets are on the horizon ahead. Use the space in between to gather your breath and take the much-needed rest before the next wave comes. Relax your jaw, release your grip, and feel yourself opening and expanding to make way for baby.

HOW TO UTILIZE A BIRTH BALL

All fours on the floor: Lean over the birth ball to help take pressure off your wrists when on all fours.

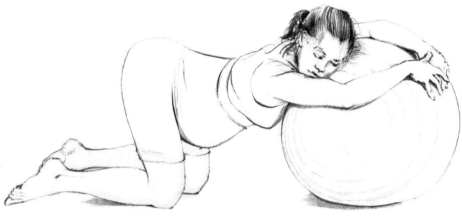

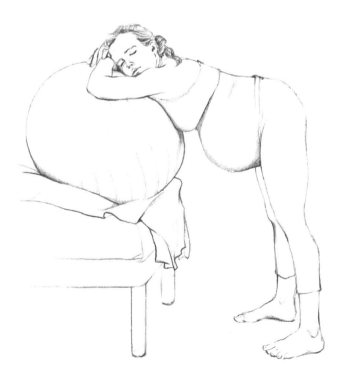

Over the bed: This is a great way to use the birth ball in the hospital. No need to get in the bed; instead, place the ball on the bed to lean on, and use gravity and movement while laboring.

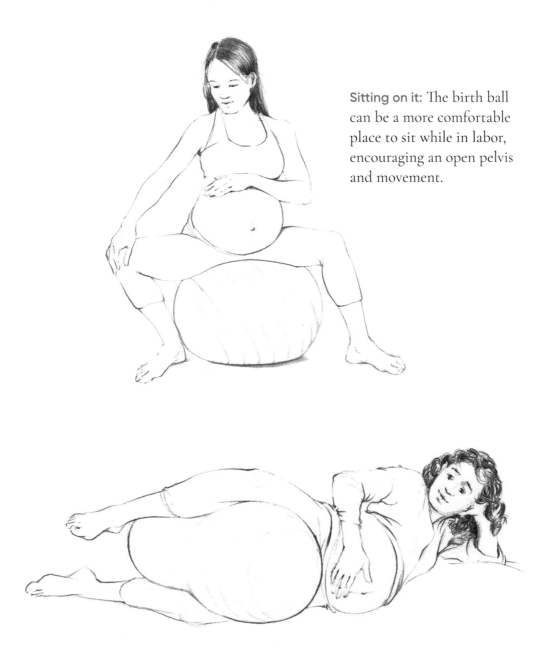

Sitting on it: The birth ball can be a more comfortable place to sit while in labor, encouraging an open pelvis and movement.

Peanut ball: The peanut ball is incredibly useful for those who choose to get an epidural in labor. It helps keep the hips open and encourages the fetal rotation necessary for birth.

DILATION STATION

Believe it or not, the toilet is a great place to labor. What happens when we sit on the toilet? Our pelvic floor knows to relax. It's the only place we are really used to allowing fluids to flow out of us. Being on the toilet also encourages a squat-like position that can help the baby's head engage and intensify contractions. I also like to use the bathroom as a private cave for parents to escape to for privacy and alone time. Straddle the toilet facing the wall and put a pillow down on the back of the toilet so you can rest your arms and head.

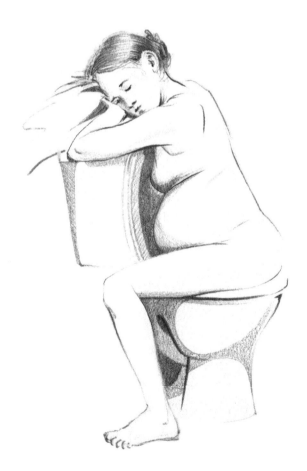

WATER BIRTH AND THE AQUADURAL

Water has been used as a method of pain relief for centuries, and several studies have shown that a water birth is associated with faster labor, less complicated births, lower likelihood of induction and Cesarean, and decreased risk of severe tearing and postpartum hemorrhage. Studies have also shown lower rates of respiratory distress and hospitalization for babies compared to those born on land at home.[71]

Whether or not you plan to give birth in the water, I highly recommend utilizing water in your labor. I have seen water work wonders as a natural pain reliever. Most labor and delivery rooms have showers, and if you're lucky, your hospital room will have a bathtub too. This is less common, but something to ask about if you are planning to have an unmedicated birth. If your birthing place doesn't offer water relief,

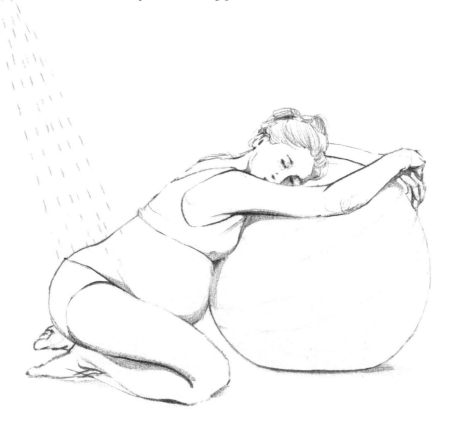

193

then all the more reason to labor at home for as long as possible so that you can use your own shower or bath. Access to water is one of the many benefits of home birth, where water can be enjoyed at any stage of labor. With that said, it is such a powerful tool that you may want to consider saving it for the moment you need it the most. Let the water run directly onto your lower back. You can also find relief with a warm water bottle or heat pad placed on your lower back or abdomen.

BREATH

Deep breathing is a wonderful tool for calming the nervous system, but I don't believe that you must learn a specific method of breathing in order to give birth. What is far more important than how you breathe is that you breathe and that you feel uninhibited to vocalize as you please. Turn back to Weeks 13 and 15 for more on this topic. Ask your partner to breathe deeply and slowly along with you. Synchronizing your breathing will help center you through co-regulating your nervous systems. The meditations in Weeks 17, 19, and 22 can also serve as inspiration.

HYPNOBIRTH

Hypnobirth is a birthing technique that promotes tools to help access a pain-free or even pleasurable birth. In my experience, hypnobirthing is most effective in helping people deprogram from the fearful and negative rhetoric around birth to help establish a mindset of trust in themselves, their baby, and the physiological process.

I once attended a birth where the mama smiled ear to ear through every single contraction to signal a positive association and bridge the mind-body connection. Studies have found that smiling during stressors can reduce the intensity of the body's stress response, regardless of whether a person feels happy. Your thoughts are more powerful than you realize and play a vital role in getting you through labor.

THE EPIDURAL AND OTHER PAIN MEDICATIONS

Many people have the misconception that doulas only support unmedicated births, but doulas are there to support women through whatever they need to birth their baby, and when it comes to birth there is not one "right" way to do it. For some avoiding medication in labor is why they hire a doula, and for others having access to an epidural along with the loving support of a doula is what is desired for a positive birth experience. For those who want complete pain relief in labor, epidurals are highly effective in reducing pain and a widely used method of pain relief. In fact, around 80 percent of women in the United States utilize an epidural in labor.[72]

I have supported a number of women who have utilized this tool for pain relief and have observed a wide range of outcomes as a result. I have seen women truly benefit from the use of an epidural and I have seen births suffer serious consequences as a result of the misuse of this intervention. So let's dive into what an epidural does, the risks and benefits, and what to expect if you choose to utilize it.

An epidural utilizes a catheter placed near the spine to deliver opioid narcotics such as fentanyl or morphine, numbing the lower part of your body from the abdomen down to the feet. The narcotics administered by the epidural drip continuously throughout the duration of labor, providing long-lasting relief until after delivery, when it is removed.

When Not to Use the Epidural

The epidural can be a helpful tool when used correctly. It is important that the decision comes from the laboring mother in response to her current need, not in anticipation of what is to come or from external pressure from doctors or anyone else around her. A prevalent myth I hear is that you only have a limited window of time to receive the

195

Epidural Pros and Cons

PROS

+ Generally, very effective in providing complete relief.

+ Allows laboring mama to get some rest if desired.

CONS

✗ Once an epidural is placed, birth becomes more medicalized as a result (continuous fetal monitoring, continuous blood pressure monitoring, and IV administration all become nonnegotiable).

✗ A catheter is placed in the urethra because you can't get up to use the bathroom.

✗ Epidurals greatly limit mobility. Movement is key for progress and fetal positioning. As a result, this can lead to cascading interventions, induction, or Cesarean.

✗ There is no long-term data that demonstrates the safety of opioid exposure in utero.

✗ The medication and procedure itself have potential side effects. One more common side effect is a chronic headache for weeks or months after birth if a nerve is hit.

✗ Epidurals are associated with a drop in blood pressure, change in baby's heart rate, fever, a longer labor (increasing likelihood of Pitocin and other interventions), and limited mobility as a result of loss of sensation.

✗ An epidural disrupts the symphony of birth hormones.

✗ Not being able to feel the urge to push can make pushing more challenging.

✗ Some studies show epidural use may interfere with early breastfeeding.

✗ Some reports express a more challenging recovery because mom is also detoxing post birth.

epidural. This is not true. There is no cut-off time where you can no longer ask for an epidural, unless, of course, your baby is coming out of you faster than it can be administered. If you choose to use an epidural, you may benefit from holding off as long as possible so that you can utilize movement before being confined to the bed.

Walking Epidural: The term walking epidural is used to describe a low-dose epidural, but the name is misleading because most people still can't walk with a "walking epidural," and even if you could, hospital staff would be far too concerned with the liability to allow you to do so. A low-dose epidural comes with most of the same benefits and risks but may allow for more sensation to aid in movement and pushing efforts.

Intravenous Narcotics (IV): Narcotics administered intravenously into the bloodstream provide temporary relief and are generally less effective than the epidural. The risks seem to outweigh the benefits because more of the medication reaches the baby in utero than a localized epidural. This can result in drowsiness and possible breathing difficulties for the newborn.[73]

Nitrous Oxide: Nitrous oxide gas is another medical drug utilized as pain management in labor. The gas is inhaled through a mask to provide relief to the entire body, without causing total loss of feeling or loss of muscle movement. It is not as effective as the epidural and wears off quickly, making it a more desirable option for those who just want temporary relief. The risks have not been widely researched, but there is some correlation between nitrous oxide use in labor and vitamin B12 deficiency in infants.

197

Birth Affirmations

When we slow down our thoughts, we can hear the wisdom
within us. When we focus our attention away from the negative
talk, fear, and doubt, we give light to our inner strength.
No matter how much birth support you have, the journey
to motherhood requires you to go inward and show up for
yourself, to believe in yourself. Birth invites you to connect with
unconditional self-love. Spend some time writing out your birth
affirmations and mantras that
will ground you in your inner voice of confidence.

EXAMPLES

EACH WAVE BRINGS ME CLOSER TO MY BABY.

THIS IS NOT BIGGER THAN ME, THIS IS ME.

MY BODY AND BABY ARE WORKING IN HARMONY.

OPEN.

WE ARE SAFE.

THE ONLY WAY OUT IS THROUGH.

Week 32

SLEEP SOLUTIONS

Sleeping comfortably through the night may be a bit of a challenge these days. Getting up to pee constantly, achy hips, and perhaps a racing mind make quality sleep hard to come by in the third trimester. Here are some tips that may help.

- Get fifteen to thirty minutes of sunshine (without sunglasses) first thing in the morning. This will support your circadian rhythm.

- Avoid being on screens at least two hours before bed. If you do use screens before bed, use blue light–blocking glasses.

- Use blackout curtains and make sure all light sources are covered.

- Have a protein-rich bedside snack that will help sustain your blood sugar through the night.

199

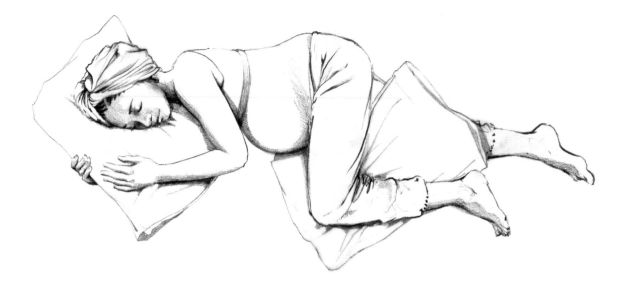

This sleep position can help alleviate discomfort in the hips for better sleep. By using pillows for support, the mother is able to rotate forward without placing too much pressure onto her belly.

- Magnesium supplements can help the body relax and ease any tension.

- Check in with how caffeine is feeling for you. Your metabolism changes in pregnancy and some people become more sensitive to it.

- Try incorporating some more movement and exercise into your day.

- Use a pregnancy pillow or position your bed pillows around you to support your hips while you sleep.

Although the physical sleep discomforts will subside after pregnancy, early motherhood comes with an entirely new set of adjustments when it comes to sleep. People are always so quick to tell expectant parents that every day of early parenthood is cursed with utter EXHAUSTION and sleep deprivation. We know that sleep is a crucial aspect of our health and ability to recover, so why, then, is sleep so hard to come by for so many new parents? While it's no secret that the first year of motherhood is likely not going to be the most restful period of your life, I have found from personal experience and through my work that you can have a new baby who doesn't sleep through the night and still feel rested. What if I told you modern parenting approaches, not babies, are to blame for the sheer level of exhaustion new parents feel?

BED-SHARING

The American Academy of Pediatrics strongly discourages bed-sharing, but risk factors are not the same for everyone. With the prevailing conversation centered around the dangers of bed-sharing the evidence-based benefits are often overlooked, and many parents are left without the proper information on doing it safely.

The Benefits of Bed-Sharing

Making the conscious choice to share a bed with our baby meant that those inevitable night wakes, diaper changes, and feeds could be done without having to get out of bed in the middle of the night. It allowed me to nurse her as needed in our sleep, and frankly, I slept better knowing she was safe right beside me. My first year of motherhood would have looked very different if not for bed-sharing, but the benefits of bed-sharing go far beyond convenience for mamas. It's biologically in the best interest of babies too. Bed-sharing is linked to immunological and neurological benefits for babies, promotes healthy milk supply, and helps regulate baby's temperature and nervous system. Co-sleeping babies imitate the breathing patterns of their parents and are more aroused through the night. When done safely, co-sleeping reduces the risk of sudden infant death syndrome. In Japan, where co-sleeping is the cultural norm, rates of SIDS are the lowest in the world.

Unsafe Bed-Sharing

Roughly half of all reports of SIDS take place while co-sleeping.[74] This is an alarming statistic that influences the guidance to avoid bed-sharing and deters many parents. However, when we break down the data, it is not as black-and-white as it is made out to seem. The fact that 92 percent of those deaths occurred under hazardous circumstances is worth pointing out. Bed-sharing is not going to be the safest option for everyone, but when we remove unsafe sleeping habits, the risks plummet. Below are some of the factors that constitute an unsafe sleep environment for baby:

- Sleeping on a couch or in a rocking chair, waterbed, or recliner.

- Sleeping in the bed with someone who uses drugs, takes sleeping pills, drinks alcohol, or smokes cigarettes.

- When there are animals or other children in the bed.

- When a parent has a medical condition that impacts their sleep.

- When there are heavy blankets and excess pillows that could suffocate. Baby should be undressed or in light clothing to prevent overheating.

- When bed-sharing with babies who are exclusively bottle-fed formula. Formula is digested differently than breast milk, and babies who are formula fed tend to stay satiated with full bellies for longer. Although this is touted as a formula perk, there are health benefits of an easily aroused baby.

Every family and baby is unique, and I recognize that bed-sharing might not be the best or safest option for everyone, but to tell all parents that it's unsafe is just not true and creates unnecessary shame. It is important for each family to decide on the sleeping arrangement that best fits their needs. There is no one-size-fits-all answer. When information on safe co-sleeping practices is withheld and replaced with fear tactics it compromises optimal rest and safety.

Safe Bed-Sharing

Prepare your sleep environment by making sure there are no gaps between the mattress and headboard or wall and that all excess bedding is removed.

When your baby is old enough to roll or crawl off the bed, you may want to consider moving your mattress to the floor.

The cuddle curl depicted below is the ideal co-sleeping position that most co-sleeping mamas naturally find themselves in. You see here that her top arm is keeping her pillow under her head and her bottom legs curl under her baby to prevent him from sinking down below the comforter. This crescent moon shape provides the perfect protective space for your baby.

203

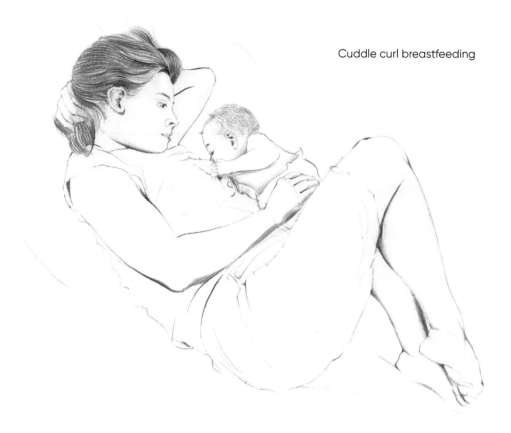

Cuddle curl breastfeeding

Bed-Sharing and Your Romance

Concerns of loss of physical intimacy after parenthood are very real and something I will continue to touch upon in the weeks to come. Parenthood, especially in the first year, can take an enormous toll on a union. Relationships are living and growing organisms that need to be continually nurtured to flourish.

Although the needs within each unique partnership are important to acknowledge, dynamics within relationships will inevitably shift after birth and that's okay. Early parenthood is a temporary season that can inspire new ways to strengthen your romantic bond and intimacy that can be even more rewarding than ever before. This may mean having to get creative. I have heard it said on more than one occasion, "Never trust the couch of a co-sleeper."

ONCE A CO-SLEEPER, ALWAYS A CO-SLEEPER?

People used to tell my parents all the reasons why they should put us in our own beds, but my grandmother would say in her loving way, "There will come a day when your babies no longer want to sleep in your bed. So just enjoy it while you can." She was right. It wasn't forever. We eventually slept in our own beds, and now I live across the country from my parents and I now bed-share with my baby. Everything has its season. I can't tell you when your child will feel ready to sleep solo, and truth be told, your readiness might not be at the same time as your child's. Some people will tell you that bed-sharing creates an unhealthy codependency, but I have found it fosters a greater sense of independence. The central theme in the attachment theory approach to parenting is that when children feel secure, they feel more confident in exploring the world. As your baby grows, you can always reassess how co-sleeping is working for you and your family and make conscious, gentle changes.

OTHER SLEEPING OPTIONS

If you don't plan to bed-share, you and your baby will still benefit from room sharing for at least the first six months of life. Room sharing reduces the rate of SIDS by 50 percent and is supportive of breast-feeding relationships. Bassinets that attach to the side of the bed are a great alternative that gives the baby his own sleeping surface nearby. What is most important is that your baby's cries are met with connection. This can take place regardless of where they sleep.

A Nightly Gratitude Ritual

Every night from as far back as I can remember my mother would tuck me into bed and invite me to say my prayers, thanking God for all that I am grateful for. She and I would recite the Lord's Prayer together, a nightly ritual her grandmother and she once shared. This is a nightly ritual that has stayed with me and one I will pass to my daughter.

When you rest your head on your pillow tonight, give thanks for all the blessings in your life and anything you are particularly grateful for this week or day.

RECONSIDERING CIRCUMCISION

The rate of circumcision is on the decline in the United States, yet circumcision is still the most frequent surgery conducted on children. It is the only operation that is regularly performed without any medical need on healthy infants. Circumcision is an ancient ritual that stems all the way back to ancient Egypt. There are many differing theories of its origin, but we know that it has been practiced over time to signify belonging to a tribe or religious group, punish prisoners of war, mark a rite of passage, condemn sexual impulses, and as a means of spiritual and hygienic purification.

In the late 1800s, Dr. John Harvey Kellogg, the founder of Kellogg's Corn Flakes and the leader of an anti-masturbation association, promoted tying the hands, electric shock therapy, caging the genitals, and circumcision to prevent a young boy from masturbating. He also believed that the pain inflicted upon the child in the circumcision

207

procedure would help instill a sense of punishment and shame that would deter any sexual inclinations.

Today in the United States, circumcision is performed on newborns for cosmetic reasons, as a religious ritual, or due to the belief that it protects against future infections.

However, an extensive review of all available literature found that there were no randomized trials on newborn circumcision that support the suggested benefits and no evidence to justify this procedure on a medical basis.

Working as a postpartum doula for a family with a newborn greatly informed my understanding of circumcision. In the hours after this child's surgery, his temperament changed completely and he was noticeably distressed, lethargic from the anesthetic, irritable, and so clearly in pain. His mother recognized his state of discomfort and gave him Tylenol, as the doctor instructed, and I found myself wondering why a mother would allow her newborn child to undergo an elective, cosmetic operation that she knew would result in enough pain to necessitate medication for the days to follow. When I changed his diaper, I was in disbelief. The tip of his penis was swollen and red and blood stained his diaper. My heart sank. If this had been done to a baby girl it would be considered genital mutilation, but for boys it's a routine cosmetic surgery that 60 percent of parents choose to partake in.

WHAT IS FORESKIN AND IS IT EVEN NECESSARY?

Foreskin is an essential part of human anatomy. It contains a concentration of blood vessels and nerve endings and is lined with muscle fibers. Much like the skin of the eyelid, it is a thin and delicate protective covering. The foreskin makes up at least 80 percent of the penile skin covering and is as sensitive as fingertips or the lips. In fact, it has a greater concentration of nerve receptors than any other part of the penis. Circumcision cuts off over 20,000 nerve endings, impacting circulation. During erection, the foreskin glides freely over the shaft, which provides more pleasure for the partner who is stimulated by the moving pressure rather than just friction.

WHAT ARE THE RISKS OF CIRCUMCISION?

The procedure does not come without risks. The rate of complications is one in five hundred, and the most common complications are bleeding, infections, and "imperfect amount of tissue removed." Roughly 10 percent of circumcised males develop meatal stenosis, a condition in which the urethra becomes abnormally narrow.

Other downsides include the severing of lymphatic vessels,[75] which may have an impact on breastfeeding and bonding in the early days and weeks of life,[76] and the unnecessary stress on the newborn from pain. Up until the 1980s, newborns did not receive pain treatment for circumcision as it was believed that they didn't experience pain in the same way older children and adults do. Research has since revealed otherwise and although anesthetics are utilized today, studies demonstrate that no treatment options completely prevented noticeable pain in response to circumcision.

HONORING RELIGIOUS BELIEFS

Coming from a Jewish family, I recognize that the Bris is an important aspect of the Jewish tradition and symbolizes the covenant between God and the Jewish people. Although I feel very connected and proud of my Jewish heritage, there are many religious practices outlined in the Hebrew Bible that I do not practice, and I know the same to be true for my Jewish friends and family. Why the religious ritual of circumcision seems to have prevailed over time while many others have fallen away, I can't answer. However, as the implications of circumcision are

209

more understood, there are a growing number of Jewish people who are adopting an alternative ritual that honors the sacredness of the Bris without the physical act of circumcision.

Many parents consider circumcision because they want to prevent their child from feeling excluded or different from their male role models and peers. The human desire to belong is strong within all of us, and going against the tribe challenges our deeply ingrained survival instincts. As a mother, I shudder at the thought of my child being teased or ridiculed for any reason, and if there were a magic wand I could wave to ensure that she would never face cruelty I would wave it all day long. The truth is, we can't always protect our children from the callousness of others, but we can provide a foundation of love and acceptance so that our children have a strong sense of self-worth and feel safe turning to us for solace. What message do we send our children when we feel the need to surgically alter their physical appearance to fit into a societal norm?

Letting Go of External Expectations

This week I invite you to reflect on what it means to you to be a part of a tribe. Where in your life do you seek approval from others? How may this impact your decision making as a parent? What are the expectations you have of yourself or that others have of you that are no longer serving you? What feelings come up for you when you go against the grain? What feelings come up for you when you go against your intuition?

THE SACRED WINDOW

With just several weeks left to go, you may be feeling that strong urge to nest and get everything ready for your baby's arrival. So often mamas put all their focus on birth and preparing for a newborn that they forget to set themselves up for the support they need in the postpartum period. Mothers are the heart of a family and when a mama is in a state of balance and well-being, it sets the tone for the entire home and everyone benefits. Babies don't care about the latest and greatest fancy gadget or toy. The only newborn essential is a mama who is well cared for so she has the capacity to give fully to her child.

I often hear the word *postpartum* being used synonymously with *postpartum depression*, but they are not the same. The postpartum period is defined as the period after a woman gives birth. Everyone who gives birth goes through the postpartum period, but not everyone goes through postpartum depression. The length of time a mother is in the postpartum period is not universally agreed upon. The Western medical model defines this period as the first six weeks after birth, but other cultures consider the postpartum period to be the first forty days or a fourth trimester (twelve to thirteen weeks). The Oxford dictionary defines *postpartum* as "following childbirth or the birth of a young," so one could argue the postpartum period is forever. After all, when we become mothers, we never return to our old selves. We are forever changed.

In Eastern traditions, the forty days after birth are referred to as The Sacred Window, a crucial time of rest and healing after birth. Across Eastern cultures we see rituals, recipes, and customs that honor the significance of postpartum healing for mothers.

The unfortunate reality is that our culture, economic model, and health care system do not recognize the importance of this time, making it very challenging for women to receive the care and rest they need. Unlike other countries that have legislation and cultural practices in place, women in the United States are not guaranteed paid leave and are often expected to "bounce back" without missing a beat. For some women the rush back to work is a choice, and for others it's a financial necessity.

Whatever your circumstances are, I invite you to plan as best you can for optimal support and rest after birth. Ask for help from friends and family, allocate a budget, and carve out all the time you can in the weeks after birth. It is not a luxury; it is a necessity. It is an investment in your future health and the well-being of your child. Instead of creating a baby registry with toys, books, and gadgets, create a registry that asks your community to invest in your postpartum period wellness. A rocking chair is not crucial to your breastfeeding journey, but access to a lactation consultant is. This concept is becoming more popular and changing the landscape of how we show up for new parents by helping them invest in what they really need.

213

I wholeheartedly believe it is possible to thrive in the postpartum period. These are the four pillars that carried me through my sacred window and allowed me to be fully present for my daughter's first weeks of life.

FOUR PILLARS OF POSTPARTUM RECOVERY

Nourishment: In earlier chapters I spoke about the importance of balanced meals for healthy blood sugar. Stable blood sugar is directly correlated to our energy level, mood, and hormone health. The postpartum period comes with a massive shift in hormones. In fact, the hormonal changes are greater than at any other time in a woman's life, including adolescence! It's no secret that what we eat impacts how we feel, but in recent years the correlation has been well documented that nutrition plays a role in our mental well-being. In fact, the author of recent study in *Lancet Psychiatry* stated, "Diet is as important to psychiatry as it is to cardiology, endocrinology, and gastroenterology."[77] Nutrient-dense, well-balanced meals (preferably in the comfort of your bed) will support lactation, hormone balance, mental health, and physical recovery.

Nourishing yourself after birth is not as simple as it sounds. With so much attention focused on feeding the baby, mamas often forget to prioritize their own nutrition. You should anticipate needing support with meals for the first six weeks at least. This may look like setting up a meal train, hiring a postpartum doula who cooks, asking a family member to help in the kitchen, or stocking the deep freezer with premade soups and easy-to-defrost homemade meals.

Choose warm cooked foods with easy-to-digest proteins and healthy fats such as avocado, ghee, butter, bone broth, braised meats, and fish, which will help with digestion. Breastfeeding burns a lot of calories, and your protein needs are even higher while breastfeeding than in pregnancy.

Aleiela's Kitchari

One of my favorite postpartum recipes is from my friend Aleiela Allen, an Ayurvedic postpartum doula. She believes that, just as our bodies know how to give birth, they also know how to heal during the post-partum period; we just need to offer our bodies tools and support to promote the natural process.

⅔ cup [130 g] red lentils (or split mung beans or red lentils)
⅓ cup [45 g] basmati rice
4 cups [960 ml] filtered water
1 Tbsp ghee or coconut oil
1 tsp ground turmeric
1 tsp ground pink Himalayan salt
¼ tsp ground cumin
1 tsp ground coriander
¼ tsp fennel seed
¼ tsp ground ginger
¼ tsp whole yellow mustard seed
Small handful fresh cilantro
1 small carrot, chopped
½ zucchini, quartered and sliced
¼ small fennel bulb, sliced
1 small beet, peeled, quartered, and sliced

Rinse the lentils and rice under running water until the water runs clear. Add to a rice cooker or pressure cooker and add fresh water.

215

Melt the ghee in a skillet over low heat and add the turmeric, salt, cumin, coriander, fennel, ginger, and mustard seed. Heat until just fragrant, 2 to 3 minutes. Add the cilantro to the pot and stir until just wilted.

Add the spice mixture, carrot, zucchini, fennel, and beet to the pressure cooker. Hit start, and have a delicious meal ready in 20 to 40 minutes.

Depending on your liking and your rice cooker, you can alter the amount of water to make kitchari thicker or more like soup.

Rest: Setting aside all obligations for the first few weeks is going to allow you to rest with the baby throughout the day as needed. This is not the time to check a bunch of things off your to-do list. Parental leave is not "vacation time." The role you are stepping into is full-time work, and if you can prioritize rest when your baby sleeps you can give your battery the recharge it needs to get through those inevitable night wakes. Be mindful of where your energy is spent and discuss with your partner who is welcome in your postpartum sanctuary and for how long. You should never feel like you are hosting others or choosing between rest and visitors. For us, having no friends or family visit until three weeks after birth allowed us to get into a rhythm and create an environment of rest and intimacy before opening our doors to others. Although this may not be the right path for every family, it was imperative for us to set that boundary.

In Week 32 I shared my thoughts on bed-sharing and how for many families it can result in greater rest. If you want to dive deeper into the topic, check out James McKenna's book *Safe Infant Sleep*. If you plan to co-sleep, you will want to have everything for night feeds and diaper changes to avoid getting out of bed or leaving the room. Don't forget a mattress protector or waterproof changing mat so you can change diapers in bed.

Whether or not you bed-share, you may want to consider dividing up shifts between you and your partner. If you are breastfeeding, then you will inevitably be up at night feeding or pumping to maintain your supply. Allowing your partner to clock a solid night's sleep so that they can rise early with baby allows mama to get a good chunk of uninterrupted morning sleep. During this time, your partner can wear the baby and prepare breakfast in bed for you upon waking. Why have two sleepy parents when you can divide and conquer?

Sleep will look different for every baby and parent, but remember this is just a temporary season. If you're not getting enough sleep, make sure that you are diligent about filling your cup with the three other pillars: nourishment, touch, and support. This will help support your adrenals and nervous system. Meditation is also a great tool to help restore and recharge with little sleep.

Touch: Giving birth is an extraordinarily strenuous physical event, and it is normal to feel tender and sore in the days and weeks that follow. Physical touch through massage and other healing modalities can be valuable not only to relax tense muscles and help heal the body, but also to support a relaxed nervous system. From utero throughout the entire span of adulthood the physical and emotional benefits of loving touch are well documented. Massage has been found to improve the function of the immune system and ward off disease by knocking down cortisol levels, the body's culprit stress hormone.

The healing nature of touch is not only delivered through professional bodywork but also attained through the embrace of a loved one. Those who experience physical contact report feeling less lonely, and research shows that a twenty-second hug or kiss can decrease cortisol levels and increase oxytocin and dopamine. Find moments of connection with your partner through touch that will ground you both.

Skin-to-skin contact with your baby is another form of restorative touch for both mama and baby, and it is associated with increased oxytocin, relaxation, and milk supply.

Support: None of these pillars is possible without support. In preparation for the postpartum period, take some time in the activity below to reflect on what support means to you and how you can set yourself up to feel held by your partner, your community, your family, and hired support. Loved ones are always eager to come visit and hold a new baby, but I believe baby cuddles must be earned. When friends and family come to visit, allow them to help around the house, fold some laundry, walk the dog, make you a tea. Don't be afraid to ask for help or to communicate what you need from them. People want to be helpful, but in a culture that lacks traditions in postpartum care, it is up to us to show them how. Before you give birth, have conversations with family members who will be in your postpartum bubble and tell them what support looks to you so that everyone has a clear understanding of expectations on all sides.

An invaluable part of my postpartum recovery was having the support of a postpartum doula who could cook nourishing meals for us and provide bodywork for me. Much like a birth doula, postpartum doulas are there to be of service to a mother so that she feels held and confident in her innate abilities to nurture her baby. In essence, what postpartum doulas do is mother the mother in whatever way she needs to be cared for.

Preparing for Postpartum Peace

Spend some time brainstorming about your postpartum care plan. Share this activity with your partner so you can start implementing a plan. This will be a helpful page to reference in the early weeks after birth.

- What does your ideal sacred window look like?

- Who in your community can you turn to for support after birth? What family members or friends can you call on?

- Who can help you organize a meal train?

- List five people in your life you can vent to without feeling judged.

- Are there any virtual or local mom groups you can join in pregnancy or the postpartum period to establish more community?

- Who would you trust to hold your baby while you receive bodywork or take a bath?

- List women in your life you can call on for guidance and encouragement around breastfeeding.

- Who can you count on to make you laugh when you need humor medicine?

- Who are the support people in your partner's life that he can turn to for support?

- What practitioners or services may be of benefit to you during the postpartum period? For example, chiropractor, masseuse, pelvic floor specialist, postpartum doula, acupuncturist, therapist, lactation consultant, etc. Gather recommendations to have on hand.

- What boundaries do you plan to implement to ensure visitors don't overstay their welcome and that you are prioritizing your family needs above all else?

BREASTFEEDING 101

In the third trimester you may start to see some colostrum leaking from your breasts. Although this can be an exciting signal that your body is getting ready to feed your little one, there is no cause for concern if you haven't spotted any yet. Your colostrum and milk will know to come when your baby arrives. Colostrum is the very first milk your body makes for baby and is rich in protein, antibodies, white blood cells, growth factor, vitamin A, zinc, and magnesium. Colostrum usually lasts a couple of days until your mature milk comes in. Now is a great time to start to gather information and resources that will support you on your breastfeeding journey to come.

BENEFITS OF BREASTFEEDING

One of the benefits of breastfeeding is that all your baby needs is within you and readily available on demand for free! However, there are some products that can be beneficial to your breastfeeding journey. The most

221

important way to set yourself up for success is to have support. Gather a list of local lactation consultants you can contact in real time. Most breastfeeding challenges arise when the mature milk comes in. Have the name of a lactation consultant at your fingertips so you can turn to a second opinion if you're not getting the proper guidance you need.

I can't emphasize enough that a great deal of patience is required for breastfeeding success. It comes as a surprise to many mamas that breastfeeding can take some work, troubleshooting, and time before it becomes a breeze. It's okay if it doesn't happen seamlessly right off the bat. If it's important to you, stick with it and surround yourself with the support you need to get through to the other side. (More on this on Week 1 Earthside.)

Sometimes breastfeeding requires a great deal of work and fortitude up front, but the payoff is well worth it. Breastfeeding has lifelong benefits for your baby and is a convenient way of nourishing her both nutritionally and emotionally. Over the years formula marketing has convinced many that breastfeeding is a burden we shouldn't have to tolerate and that formula is more convenient than breastfeeding, but the steps it takes to prepare and clean bottles is far more labor intensive than feeding from the breast. Between air travel, night wakes, tumbles, and tears, breastfeeding has been the single most convenient and effective tool I have for parenting an infant and toddler. Health benefits for baby aside, it is one of the most cherished aspects of motherhood for me.

COOL FACTS ABOUT BREAST MILK

- Your body knows to produce more water in your milk supply on hot days and more fat on cold days, creating the perfect water/fat balance for your baby.

- As babies breastfeed, they send information to their mothers about the unique needs of their immune system. Your breast milk contains customized antibodies that help your baby fight off bacteria and viruses present in your environment.

- Breastfeeding lowers the risk of babies developing asthma, allergies, or diabetes.

- Research suggests breastfed babies tend to have higher IQs.

- Breastfeeding stimulates oxytocin, which helps contract the uterus back to its regular size.

- Research shows breastfeeding reduces your risk of breast and ovarian cancers.

- Breastfeeding is ready made, free of charge, and doesn't require extra washing of bottles.

- Breastfeeding reduces the risk of SIDS.

- Breast milk contains beneficial bacteria to coat your baby's gut and promote a health microbiome.

WHAT TO HAVE ON HAND

- ☐ Firm breastfeeding pillow
- ☐ Silver nursing cups
- ☐ Glass bottles and preemie small nipple heads to slow the flow if bottle feeding
- ☐ Breast pump
- ☐ Breast milk collector
- ☐ Pumping and nursing bras
- ☐ Nursing pads
- ☐ Tincture to support healthy ducts and supply (I love WishGarden)
- ☐ Silicone ice trays and bags for freezer storage

FACTORS THAT PROMOTE BREASTFEEDING SUCCESS

- + Oxytocin
- + Skin-to-skin contact immediately after birth and as much as possible in the weeks to follow
- + SUPPORT!
- + Proper hydration and nourishment
- + Bed-sharing
- + Unmedicated birth
- + Partner encouragement
- + Feeding on demand
- + Chiropractic and craniosacral bodywork for mama and baby

FACTORS THAT CAN LIMIT BREASTFEEDING SUCCESS

- ✖ Predatory formula marketing and messaging
- ✖ Poor medical guidance
- ✖ Having a night nurse
- ✖ Bottle feeding too early
- ✖ Introducing formula
- ✖ Lack of encouraging support or community
- ✖ Unaddressed tongue tie
- ✖ Separation from baby
- ✖ Nipple shields
- ✖ Rigid feeding schedule
- ✖ Cesarean birth
- ✖ Birth trauma
- ✖ Unmanaged maternal stress
- ✖ Dehydration

Write a Letter to Your Postpartum Self

Picture yourself a few weeks or months from now after you have given birth to your baby and to the mother within. Write to this new mother as you would a friend or sister. Tell this future version of yourself how proud you are of her and what her body is capable of. Tell this new mama what you think she needs to hear as she navigates so much newness. Remind this version of yourself that she is strong, resilient, and capable. Be the cheerleader she needs. Seal it and store it away or give it to a friend to give to you during your postpartum period.

YOUR BIRTH, YOUR WAY

At thirty-six weeks of pregnancy, my client Molly called to tell me her baby was breech. She was planning a home birth with an autonomous midwife who had a great deal of experience and trust in supporting breech delivery. We talked through all her options, and she said, "I feel good going forward with my plan to birth at home. I trust my baby's wisdom; my body and I feel well supported by my birth team."

In most states, licensed midwives are not legally permitted to support breech delivery at home. Breech delivery has become somewhat of a lost art because it is no longer taught in medical school. As a result, most OBs refuse to assist in breech delivery, making Cesarean delivery prior to the onset of labor the default "option" for most women. For this reason, when babies present breech in the final weeks of pregnancy it can cause a great deal of stress for a mother birthing within a system that won't recognize her right to choose. Those final sacred weeks of pregnancy are often spent attempting to spin her baby through several interventions and routines. Sometimes it's successful, sometimes not.

There are gentle ways to encourage your baby to find his way head down, like playing music toward your lower abdomen, acupuncture, and Spinning Babies movement. Your provider may also recommend an external cephalic version (ECV), where he or she attempts to manually flip the baby by manipulating the uterus. This can be very uncomfortable and does pose risks. It is only effective about 60 percent of the time. The bottom line is that a breech-presenting baby should not rule out a vaginal birth. Although breech presentation may increase risks, Cesarean birth also contains risks. Your provider's limitations are not your limitations. It will, however, mean having to put in more effort to find a provider who is skilled and confident in supporting you.

By thirty-six weeks, 97 percent of babies will find their way head down, but the small percent of babies who choose to stay upward have their own wisdom that is simply a variation of normal. I like to remind my clients that some babies just want to stay snuggled up near the comforting rhythmic beating of their mother's heartbeat.

When Molly gave birth at forty-one weeks, we were all surprised to welcome her baby boy headfirst. He had flipped himself in labor and was born peacefully at home.

GROUP BETA STREP

This week you will be tested for group B strep, a bacteria found in the vagina of roughly 20 percent of pregnant women. When this strain of bacteria comes in contact with a baby during birth for an extended period of time, it can increase the risk of a rare but serious illness called GBS disease. In the United States, the standard of care when group B is present is to administer IV antibiotics during labor to prevent infection in newborns. Without antibiotics, 1 to 2 percent of infants develop this disease, and that number drops to 0.02 percent when antibiotics are given at least four hours prior to delivery.[78] Although antibiotics can be effective in minimizing complications, they also have their drawbacks. Antibiotics can wipe out beneficial bacteria and alter the infant microbiome, lead to allergic reactions, contribute to antibiotic resistance, and increase the risk of allergies, eczema, asthma, and diabetes.

Although the overall risk of complications from GBS disease is low, the risk is higher for those born prior to thirty-seven weeks and when the amniotic sac has been ruptured for more than eighteen hours before the baby is born. For this reason, some with GBS choose to see how their labor plays out and weigh their individual risks before deciding on an approach. Regardless of the route you choose to take, the presence of GBS does not rule out birthing at home, nor should it impact how you birth in a hospital.

PREPARING THE PERINEUM?

With just a few weeks to go you may be wondering whether there is something you should be doing now to help minimize the chance of vaginal tearing in birth. Our bodies are designed for birth and when the physiological process is supported, the slow and gradual emerging of your baby's head will do its job of stretching your perineum. It is also important to note that there is so much more at play than just the surrounding vaginal tissue alone. In Week 15, pelvic floor therapist Allison Oswald shared some techniques for engaging with the pelvic floor in preparation for birth. Focus your attention on the relaxation of the pelvic floor muscles. You may find that inserting your fingers into your vagina will give you feedback so you can feel how your breath correlates with the softening of these muscles.

Your greatest protection from severe tearing is a provider with a low episiotomy rate. An episiotomy, where the perineum is cut with

228

scissors, often results in more severe tearing and damage. Receiving an episiotomy has less to do with your vagina's capacity to expand and more to do with your provider's harmful habits. Have a conversation with your doctor or midwife prior to birth and find out how and whether they utilize this procedure, if at all. Your provider should be willing to be patient and refrain from directing you to push against your instincts or intervening unnecessarily.

Ample skin elasticity will support your perineum too. Up your intake of collagen-rich foods and foods with high vitamin C. You can also apply pure vitamin E oil to the perineum daily for greater hydration.

Purge Writing

This week's activity is geared toward releasing fears, stress, and that which no longer serves you. Take out a piece of paper and for eight minutes put pen to paper and purge write. Dump onto the page anything that is weighing you down or stressing you out. Don't worry about forming complete sentences, just WRITE IT OUT and get it onto the page. When the eight minutes are up, put your pen down. Now find a safe place to set fire to this page and allow it to burn.

BABYPROOFING YOUR RELATIONSHIP

As a self-proclaimed birth book junkie, I have read more books on pregnancy, birth, and parenthood than you could imagine! When I became a parent, I felt very prepared in most areas but soon realized that one very important topic was consistently left out of the conversation: babyproofing the relationship.

One in five couples separate within the first year of having a baby, and 65 percent of parents report dissatisfaction within their relationship, yet no one seems to be talking about it. With a nationwide divorce rate of over 50 percent, many of us didn't have healthy relationships to look up to. Whatever strains are on your partnership now will not go away when your baby arrives, and no matter how strong your foundation is as a couple, parenthood will present you with new challenges.

231

With those challenges comes an opportunity to deepen your bond, communication, and intimacy to continue to grow together.

The birth of a child comes with it the birth of parents who are figuring out their new existence in real time alongside their baby. Within a marriage or partnership there are the needs of each individual, the needs of the family, and the needs of the relationship itself. From one day to the next we are thrown into a completely new triad and expected to know how to find balance and give energy to all parts.

As a Scorpio, I am not afraid of conflict and to move on from a disagreement I need to hash things out and come to a resolution, no matter how long it takes. Let's just say, I am not one to sweep things under the rug, and my relentless efforts to get to the root of things have for the most part strengthened our communication over the seven years prior to parenthood. As soon as we became parents, I found that my default problem-solving approach was no longer serving me, nor us. I felt completely drained by drawn-out discord. Turns out, parenthood even changes the way you fight!

The most challenging days of motherhood for me are not due to sleepless nights or our daughter's temperament but have everything to do with how Johnathan and I come together. When we are united, everything parenthood throws our way feels manageable, but when we're stuck in a couple-rut nothing comes easy. For the first time I understood the advice of putting your relationship before your children. Prior to parenthood I wrote this off as selfish, but now I realize that we are better parents to our daughter and she benefits when we are well regulated and strong in our bond. Parenthood propels you to reevaluate that which no longer serves you. With the carefully observing eyes and ears of a new baby, I felt immense pressure to model loving communication, patience, and harmony at all times, which is just an unrealistic expectation.

"MOVE ON" MENTALITY

My friend Katie, a mom of two, told me that the best parenting advice she ever received was to address the issue and then move on. When her four-year-old son acts out, she is firm in her response and then lets it go, showing him that it's okay to draw boundaries, it's okay to voice a need or express disappointment, and then we forgive and continue on. We don't have to get stuck in it, and we don't have to dwell on it. This sage parenting advice is also sage relationship advice. Adopting a move on mentality doesn't mean ignoring anyone's feelings or neglecting to work on the relationship, but rather being mindful of what is worth taking up energy and space. This means becoming more efficient in your fighting, learning to let the small things go, and committing to revisiting the big things later when you are not wrapped up in emotion. Easier said than done, but if I can get there, so can you.

Co-regulation is the way that the nervous system of one individual influences the nervous system of another. We often talk about co-regulation in regard to the mother-baby dyad, but co-regulation can and should also take place within a romantic relationship. Co-regulation should not be mistaken for codependency or negating self-responsibility. Instead, it is a healthy tool for secure relationships to nurture one another in feeling grounded and centered. Parenting can be hard on the nervous system and dysregulation ripples through a family unit. When you sense your partner is stressed out and snappy, consider what they might need to feel better and ask them to do the same for you when you're in a disregulated state. Instead of reacting negatively to unpleasant vibes, rise above and let them borrow your steady nervous system.

We all fall short of the glory at times and will not always be our best selves in front of our children and that's okay. If your children see you argue, make sure they also see you come together and repair.

233

Tending to the Family Nervous System

PART ONE • **TAKE INVENTORY**

Although it's impossible to fully anticipate what you will need from your partner and what your partner will need from you in parenthood, there are things you can begin to communicate and practice now that will serve you on the other side. Maybe you notice that your partner seems less stressed after an hour at the gym or that you are in a better mood after a long bath. Notice when your nervous system feels most at peace and plan to bring these elements into your relationship. Return to this throughout the evolution of your journey. This is a living framework that will inevitably change with time.

- Discuss with one another how you anticipate needing support from one another after the baby comes.

- What do you anticipate being a challenge?

- What do you need to fill your cup?

- What does your partner need to fill their cup?

- What roles within your relationship do you anticipate will change after parenthood?

- What does your relationship need?

- What fears do you have surrounding your changing relationship?

- How can you help your partner regulate? How can they help you regulate?

- In what areas will you need to outsource support so that your needs can be met?

PART TWO • CREATE OR REVISIT YOUR VOWS

Whether or not you are married, I invite you to create (or revisit) vows to one another. Use these vows as an opportunity to set intentions for how you want to show up for one another through the highest of the highs and the lowest of the lows.

EMBRACING
A NEW PACE

In Week 30 I shared all about medical inductions, but what about "natural induction"? Expecting mamas who are eager to get labor started often ask me what they can do to "naturally" get things going at home. Sure, there's a laundry list of things you can try, but there is really nothing natural about forcing labor to happen before your baby is ready. Labor is prompted by a protein released by the baby when he or she is ready for life outside the womb. These DIY attempts to induce at home are considered harmless and gentle methods of induction within the natural birth community. However, when we attempt to rush the process, we are falling into the exact same mindset as a medical provider who is encouraging induction for no medical reason. Castor oil is perhaps the most effective in stimulating contractions at home, but it can lead to the same cascade of interventions we see with Pitocin if the cervix has not ripened. Often natural induction methods leave mama feeling exhausted in her efforts and defeated for not actively bringing labor on successfully. Patience is one of the greatest lessons parenthood affords us. Lean into it. This time is expanding you capacity for slowing down and embracing a new pace of life on the other side.

WELCOMING A SIBLING

If you're welcoming your second baby, you may be anticipating what it will feel like being a mother of two! Chances are, the soon-to-be big sibling who is also at the precipice of a big life change is also wondering how this new role will feel. Though you have been through a version of this before, no two births or babies are ever the same, so it is normal to have big feelings arise as you anticipate the balance of mothering two children at once. It is also very common for older siblings to feel this exciting shift on the horizon. They too may have some fear about what this change might mean for them and life as they know it.

No matter how young your child is, talk to them about what is to come and give them the opportunity to express all their feelings without shame or judgment. As an older sister, I can remember these mixed feelings when my little brother was born. It didn't take long for me to realize that his existence was the single best thing my parents ever did for me. Riding through life with him is the ultimate gift.

Here are some tips for helping a big brother or sister welcome a new baby into the family.

- In Week 23 I talk about the importance of celebrating a mama through her rite of passage to help integrate this big life change. Perhaps create a ritual or ceremony of recognition for your older child to make him feel valued in his new role.

237

- For some, having their older children be a part of the birth process can be very special. If you choose to welcome your child to be at your birth, prepare them for what it might look and sound like.

- If your older child is not at the birth, you may want to have your new baby out of your arms when you introduce them to one another.

- Have your new baby come with a special gift or note for her big sibling.

- Have a basket of special toys that your older one gets to play with while you are breastfeeding your newborn.

Make an Emotional Checklist

This week's activity is by my dear friend and doula mentor Lori Bregman, who has taught me so much and been a guiding light to thousands of parents.

FROM LORI

Oftentimes, during pregnancy unexpected physical, emotional, or spiritual issues rise to the surface. They may feel uncomfortable at first, but they can help you prepare for your new role as a mom and be a better parent to your child. Some examples might be challenges of patience, issues of trust, or feelings of insecurity or self-judgment. Take a moment to answer the questions below.

- What is showing up for you right now?

- How could this be preparing you for motherhood?

- How is this an opportunity to practice modeling self-love for your child?

MAKE AN EMOTIONAL CHECKLIST

List five ways you are prioritizing your well-being now and in the first few weeks of parenthood. What are five things that instantly lift your mood?

ACTIVATE YOUR RIGHT BRAIN

As you move into your final days or weeks of pregnancy, I want you to take a moment to acknowledge all of the growth you have done in every sense of the word. Week by week you have opened your mind to so much new information and have so bravely opened your heart to deep inner work and reflection to prepare for birth and motherhood. From this day forward I want you to put aside the checklists and resist the urge to do any more mental or physical preparation. Everything you need is already within you.

So much of what we do to prepare for birth uses our left brain. We think, analyze data and time, read books, take classes, etc., etc. Birth happens in our right brain, the part of our brain that is creative and primal, not from the prefrontal cortex thinking brain. In the next couple weeks, while at the precipice of transformation, this book will focus solely on activities that speak to your creative inner self, whatever that looks like for you. Spend time in nature, sleep in, do absolutely nothing, soak up solo time with yourself or your beloved, paint, draw, bake, dance, skinny-dip, and enjoy the potency of this transitional time.

Vision Candle: Pull out the old magazines and pick up a prayer candle. Instead of making a vision board, make a vision candle. Attach words and images that inspire you onto a candle using Mod Podge and meditate on your intentions for birth and motherhood each time you light your candle.

Paint the Sunset: Set up a canvas on your patio or a place nearby where you can see the sunset. Paint the sunset as a birthday gift for your baby. Don't worry about your artistic "skills." Use this as an opportunity to let go of perfectionism in preparation to flow through birth.

Bath Ritual: Draw a warm bath with Epsom salts, wildflower petals, and dried lavender. Light a candle, turn on a relaxing playlist, and brew some tea. Soak leisurely and give yourself a loving body scrub massage, letting each stroke wash away your tension and anything you want to leave behind before you enter the birth portal.

FACING THE UNKNOWN

Forty weeks is a feeling hard to describe! You're eagerly anticipating all that's to come. You've made it to what is considered the "finish line" or full term, but you still may have days or weeks to go. It is bittersweet. Pregnancy is coming to an end soon, which means you will be holding your little one in your arms any day now. It is exciting and a bit nerve-racking—it was for me at least. I knew I was about to face the deep unknown and that the only way out was through. I just wanted to get it over with already and at the same time I just wanted to stay pregnant forever.

The forty-week mark landed on my twenty-ninth birthday. Birthday calls and messages rolled in accompanied by lots of "baby yet?" texts. I knew that the likelihood of giving birth on this day was small, but still I felt defeated, like labor would surely never come! I will never forget the text I got from my sister Jennifer, who wrote, "Enjoy the last few days of being one with your baby. Soon you will have to share her with the world."

She was so right. As eager as I was to hold her in my arms and look into her eyes, birth would be the start of her journey here on Earth as her own individual being. My job would remain in place to help her grow and care for her, but she would come into her own body and live out her own destiny. Perhaps labor is so challenging because on a subconscious level we are trying to hold on to this union that will never be the same. It is inevitable, and when the time comes you have no choice but to let go and trust that the world will treat her as kindly as you have. You no longer get to breathe for her. She will soon be taking her own breaths and steps and with every passing day she will need you a little bit less.

Manifesting Your Dream Birth

So often I observe women resist allowing their minds and hearts to fully visualize what their perfect birth would look like. I must admit, I had some blocks around doing this myself. Perhaps it's superstition, not feeling worthy of the experience you desire, or the fear of disappointment if things don't go as planned that keeps us from envisioning our dream birth. Here I want to give you permission to embrace your vision fully. Be as detailed as possible about how you see your birth unfolding. It's okay to set your mind and your heart to it. It's okay to believe it's possible for birth to be everything you imagined and more. It's also okay to dream big and it's okay to feel let down if things don't go the way you imagined.

This week's journal activity is to go beyond the Birth Intentions document you previous created in Week 28 and visualize, draw, or write out your dream birth. What does it look like, smell like, feel like? Who is there to support you? How do you feel? What mindset do you embody? What intentions do you want to set for yourself of how you approach this day?

THE SPACE BETWEEN WORLDS

Well, you may feel like you have been and will be pregnant foreverrrr. I promise you, you won't be. Soon your body will no longer be your baby's habitat, but her cells have migrated to your tissues, organs, blood, and brain, where they will be carried within you for decades to come. You may also find comfort in knowing that studies have correlated higher cognitive scores in children with a longer gestation. Bonus week means bonus brain cells! Try not to watch the clock tick. Instead, pass the time soaking up the gifts from Mother Nature: stargazing, finding faces in the clouds, sitting by the shore and watching the waves come and go. Put a prayer in a glass bottle and send it off to sea or bury a time capsule that you dig up with your child in the years to come. Another fun activity is to ask your friends to send you two songs: (1) an upbeat

245

dance song and (2) a mellow jam. Make two playlists, dance your heart out, and then chill. These playlists will come in handy in labor too!

You can find my labor playlist at www.carson-meyer.com.

SIGNS AND SYNCHRONICITY

In 1920, psychologist Carl Jung coined the term *synchronicity* to explain a meaningful relationship between two events that could not be explained by cause and effect. An example of this is thinking about someone you haven't seen in years and then running into them by surprise moments later in the grocery store, or when you overhear a conversation that contains the answer to something you've been internally contemplating.

During my pregnancy, I saw hearts everywhere I turned. The milk in my tea, the clouds in the sky, sidewalk chalk drawings, and fallen leaves all seemed to take the shape of a heart. I preserved these signs as messages and guidance from my baby.

Skeptics may say these coincidences can be explained by confirmation bias, the underlying tendency to notice, focus on, and give greater credence to evidence that fits with our existing belief. Regardless of what you believe, you can observe the patterns in front of you to help direct your focus in the direction you want to go. Where you place your awareness is where your energy travels. Mindfulness practices help you slow down and observe what is in front of you. It fosters a feeling of interconnectedness with the universe.

Chicken Seaweed Soup

This recipe is by my lovely postpartum doula Bella Bailey and inspired by a Chinese postpartum soup my grandmother's best friend, Audrey, would make for new mothers in her life to support hormones in the postpartum period. It is easy to make and keep frozen for after birth. One of the best ways to plan ahead is to stockpile nutritious meals in your freezer. This is one that stores well and is incredibly nourishing.

1 whole chicken
8 to 10 cups [1.9 to 2.4 L] water or chicken broth
   (homemade broth recipe on page 51)
1 onion, chopped
1 Tbsp grated fresh ginger
2 cups [400 g] dried seaweed
1 Tbsp tamari
1 tsp salt

Place the chicken in a large pot and cover completely with the water. Bring the water to a boil over high heat, and then lower the heat to maintain a simmer. Simmer over low heat for 1 hour. Add the onion, ginger, and seaweed and simmer for 2 to 3 hours longer.

Remove the chicken from the pot and shred the meat into a bowl. Return the shredded chicken to the pot and add salt and tamari.

Signs & Synchronicities

This week, in your journal, reflect on some of the synchronicities in your life and whether they have played a part in guiding you. As you go about your week, find a moment of stillness to take inventory of the directions in which your thoughts flow and how you can reroute them to bring more light and positivity to your life.

Jot down any questions you want to ask the universe or your baby and notice how the answers come to you.

TRAVELING THROUGH TIME

Think back to a year ago from today. Where were you? Who were you? What were your biggest tigers at the time? What were you feeling most impatient about? Write a letter to the version of you 365 days ago. The version of you that was not yet pregnant. Look how far you've come. Tell her how her life has changed and what she has learned along the way. Looking back on the previous year, what are you grateful for? How did you play an active role in co-creating these blessings? It may feel like you've been waiting for your baby to arrive into your arms forever, but before you know it another 356 days will come and go and you will look back at the woman you are today and tell her . . . the happiest days of her life are just around the corner.

249

THE SEA & THE MOON
DANCE TOGETHER
FORMING WAVES THAT
SHAPE THE SHORE.
WITHIN YOU LIES THE SALT
OF THE SEA,

THE STARS IN THE SKY,
THE GLOW OF THE MOON,
AND THE WARMTH
OF THE SUN.
YOU ARE MOTHER EARTH,
A CREATOR, A SYMPHONY
IN PERFECT HARMONY
WITH THE ECOSYSTEM
THAT IS YOU.

MAY YOU TRUST IN
THE DIVINE CULMINATION
THAT BROUGHT YOU HERE.
MAY YOU HOLD CLOSE
YOUR POWER AND HONOR
THE WISDOM THAT,
LIKE A WAVE,
HAS TRAVELED MILLIONS
OF YEARS TO REACH YOU.

I WILL MEET YOU
ON THE OTHER SIDE…

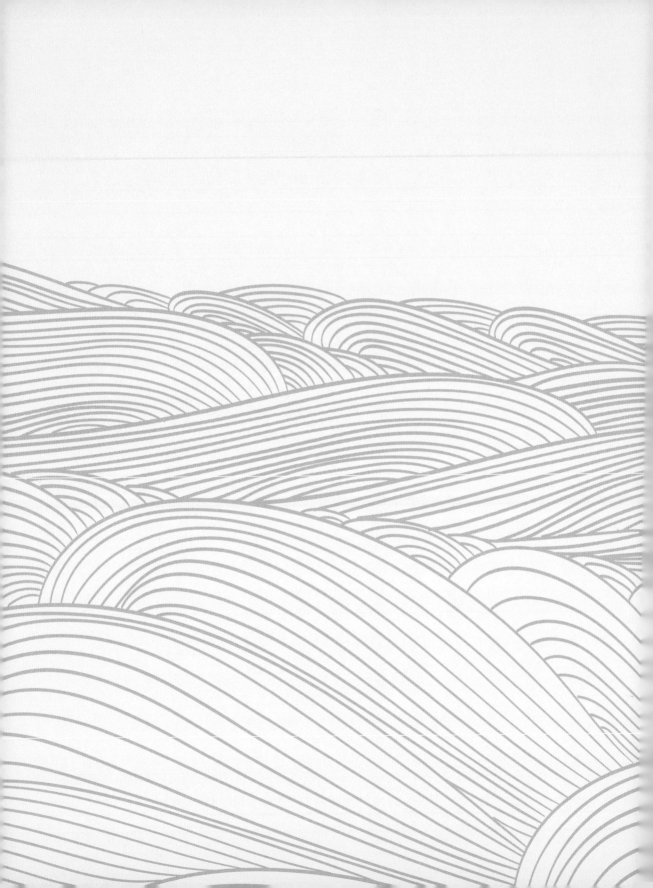

The First 100 Days

FOURTH TRIMESTER

"You are the bows from which your
children as living arrows are sent forth.

The archer sees the mark upon the path
of the infinite, and He bends you with His might
that His arrows may go swift and far.

Let your bending in the archer's hand be for gladness;

For even as He loves the arrow that flies,
so He loves also the bow that is stable."

KHALIL GIBRAN

REBIRTHED

Congratulations and welcome to the other side! You did it! What a whirlwind of blissful love you must be in and perhaps some tears and hemorrhoids too. Have grace for yourself as you feel all the different emotions that come and go. You crossed a life-changing threshold, you transformed from maiden to mother. It is big work, it's holy work, and you're doing it! You ushered a soul through the portal to Earth, which is why this chapter is called "Earthside." You have birthed a human being, parents, and a family. You journeyed to another dimension to guide your baby through and claimed a new part of yourself. No matter how your birth experience unfolded, I know you accessed an utmost level of strength to get your baby here.

I hope you are taking it easy in bed with good nourishment, support, and lots of skin-to-skin baby cuddles. If it's warm enough outside, don't forget to get some morning sunshine for you and baby. Fresh air and sunshine are not just an instant mood lifter but also an excellent source of vitamin D. Studies have shown that jaundice levels are lower in newborns with optimal vitamin D levels.[79]

HEALING AND BREASTFEEDING

After the comedown of the greatest high, you may be starting to feel more tenderness and swelling. Whether you gave birth vaginally or by Cesarean, your body has worked hard to bring your baby earthside. Rest and nourishment are essential for healing. If you have any vaginal tearing it is important that you keep your legs together as much as possible and limit your movement to allow the tissues to heal and come back together. If you didn't tear you may be feeling soreness and microtears from the stretched tissue that need some time to heal. Something that was so helpful for me in the early days was to master the side-lying feed.

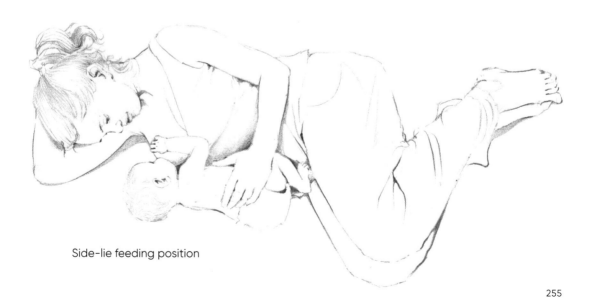

Side-lie feeding position

255

This allows you to be off your tailbone while breastfeeding. If feeding upright feels best for you, spend time lying down in between feeds to prevent putting too much pressure on your tailbone and perineum. They also make round donut-shaped seat cushions that can alleviate discomfort from sitting, which is especially helpful if you have any tearing.

If you gave birth via Cesarean, you may find the "football hold" to be the most comfortable position for breastfeeding while your incision heals. This allows you to hold baby at your breast without coming too close to the sensitive abdominal area or incision. It's also a great position for breastfeeding twins.

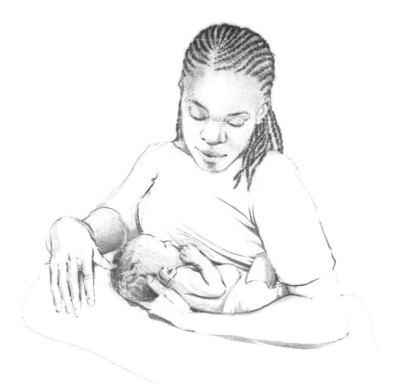

The football hold feeding position can be extra supportive for nursing twins or post-Cesarean nursing to keep baby off mom's abdomen.

OTHER TIPS FOR HEALING

Here are some other tips for healing in the first week or two post birth.

Peri Bottle: Keep a peri bottle of water by the toilet and spray it toward your urethra as you urinate. This will dilute the urine to prevent the acidity from stinging any abrasions. It will also help keep the area clean. You can add a pinch of salt and/or a couple of drops of lavender essential oil to promote healing and cleansing.

Homeopathic Oral Arnica: Homeopathic oral arnica can be placed under the tongue immediately after birth to help reduce pain. Homeopathic arnica can also be used to support healing after vaginal or Cesarean birth as needed with no known side effects. Homeopathy has been unutilized traditionally for decades and is considered safe for pregnancy and breastfeeding.

Witch Hazel: Lochia is the blood and uterine tissue that passes for a few weeks after giving birth. It can come and go and tends to become gradually lighter over time. You will want to have plenty of large organic menstrual/maternity pads on hand and change your pad frequently. You can apply witch hazel (without alcohol) to a fresh pad to reduce inflammation and swelling.

Herbal Sitz Bath: This is especially helpful for sensitive tissues.

In a small pot, bring 4 cups [960 ml] of water to a boil, then turn off the heat.

Add 2 Tbsp each of organic dried lavender, chamomile flower, and yarrow. These herbs are known for their anti-inflammatory,

257

soothing, and wound-healing properties. Stir and let sit until well steeped (10 to 20 minutes).

Using a tea strainer, carefully strain the liquid into a measuring cup and let cool. This is now your herbal sitz bath tea.

You can add this to your bathtub with warm water or pour it into a sitz bath that can be placed above your toilet basin.

Padsicles: Cool padsicles can feel really soothing and help reduce swelling around the vagina. However, cold, moist environments are not always conducive to healing tissues, so they should not be worn for extended periods of time. Once the pad no longer provides cool relief, remove it.

Unfold the pads (keeping them attached to the wrapper) on a clean, flat surface. Spray the pad lightly with witch hazel and pour 1 Tbsp or so of the herbal sitz bath tea onto each pad. The pad should not be completely soaked, just lightly moistened.

Rewrap the pads in the same wrapper or rewrap them in wax paper. Place in a zip-top bag and store in the freezer.

To use, place the padsicle in your underwear or, better yet, in an organic adult diaper (to prevent them from leaking).

Hemorrhoids: You may have experienced hemorrhoids in pregnancy or perhaps they came about for the first time as a result of your pushing efforts. Although they will get better with time, there are things you can do to help the healing progress more quickly. Potato poultices have been used for hundreds of years to draw out infection, reduce inflammation, and promote wound healing.

Wash and remove the skin from a raw russet potato.

Grate the potato and wrap it in cheesecloth.

Place a towel on the bed or comfortable surface where you can lie on your side. Firmly place the grated potato enclosed in cheesecloth into the area.

Try to keep it there for at least 20 minutes, and up to 1 to 2 hours if possible, for best results.

Cesarean Healing: Some healing practices after a Cesarean may look different but the most important elements of postpartum healing remain true: rest, nourishment, and support are essential. Remember, Cesarean birth is a major abdominal surgery, and the recovery is often more challenging than the recovery from a vaginal birth. Be mindful not to lift anything heavier than your baby and to keep hydrated to alleviate any swelling caused from the medications. You may also want to consider taking probiotics to aid in digestion and support healthy bacteria in your breast milk after antibiotics use.

Many women find belly wraps supportive after vaginal and Cesarean birth to help reengage with core muscles. You will also want to allow the area to air out while healing.

After your incision has healed, spend some time each day gently and lovingly massaging your scar with warm oil to help break up scar tissue. This can be done after or before one of the meditations or activities in Week 19 (Second Trimester) and Week 4 (Earthside) of the book. Touch is a powerful way to reconnect with your body while recognizing all that it has gone through.

MOM'S DREADED FIRST POOP

The first bowel movement after birth can be scary and probably the last thing you want to think about in the tender days postpartum. Here are some tips to help support the digestive flow with ease.

259

- Take a deep breath, be patient, and try not to avoid a bowel movement. This can contribute to constipation.

- Drink lots of water with lemon juice and warm fluids, such as raspberry leaf, ginger, and jujube tea.

- Focus on warm foods that are easy to digest. Homemade bone broth, soups, and oatmeal with coconut milk, chia seeds, prunes, berries, plum or peach, and healthy fats will help lubricate the digestive tract.

- Magnesium citrate is the form of magnesium that can cause stool to become loose. Opt for at least 350 mg per day.

- Take 1,600 mg of slippery elm bark powder mixed in water before bed.

BREASTFEEDING

The first few days postpartum your body is producing colostrum until your milk comes in at around two to five days after birth. In these early days it may not seem like there is much coming out and that is by design. At this stage your baby's stomach is about the size of a cherry and the nutrient density of colostrum means a little goes a long way. By next week your baby's tummy will grow to the size of an apricot to accommodate the increase in milk to come.

HOW DO I KNOW IF MY BABY IS GETTING ENOUGH MILK?

Wet diapers are a good indication that your baby is being well hydrated. You want to see at least one poop on the first day, two poops on the second day, and three poops on the third day. As baby nurses, listen to the sound they make and see if you notice a gulp and can see moist milky lips post feed. An underfed baby will communicate hunger through abnormal lethargy or excess irritability. Your mama wisdom will know if your baby is not getting enough. Never hesitate to reach out to a lactation consultant if you have concerns.

Remember that the quantity of your milk is based on supply and demand. The more you feed, the more your body will supply. Frequent feeding and/or pumping is essential for maintaining supply. One of the main reasons new mothers see a drop in milk supply is because they are told their baby needs more milk and they begin to supplement with formula. In doing so, they may skip breastfeeding, which further decreases supply.

HOW LONG SHOULD EACH FEED BE?

I'm not big on placing time expectations or limits on mamas and babies. We are all unique and there are so many different factors at play. Some babies cluster feed small amounts frequently and others take on larger amounts less frequently. Some babies have a very strong and efficient suck, while others may need more time at the breast to fill their tummy. This also depends on the speed of mama's milk flow.

Allowing your baby to feed for as long as she needs and as often as desired is going to optimize baby's growth and your milk supply. The breast should be readily available to your baby throughout the day and night to maintain supply. Unless there are medical concerns regarding weight gain, there is no reason to wake a sleeping baby to feed. Your baby is wise and deeply in tune with her needs. Follow her lead.

DO I NEED TO SWITCH BREASTS EACH FEED?

Some women switch breasts each feed and others switch in the middle of a feed. This will depend on how long your baby feeds for. The milk that is in the front is called foremilk and it has a higher water content to

261

provide ample hydration. The milk behind the foremilk is called hindmilk, which is a fattier milk. Allowing your baby to empty your breast completely will encourage him to get that fatty hindmilk and prevent you from getting clogged ducts. If you don't switch during a feed, be sure to switch on the next feed so that you encourage supply on both sides.

Once your milk comes in, you may feel like your breasts are always full! Things will balance out over the coming weeks. If you have an oversupply, try not to pump too often because you may overstimulate and create an even greater supply. Hand expressing or using a collection pump such as the Hakka can help you gather excess milk for the freezer and empty the breast without overstimulating.

HELP! MY NIPPLES HURT!

The first twenty-four hours of breastfeeding were a breeze for me and then on day two my milk came in and my breasts swelled up like giant balloons. My nipples were chapped and hurt like hell! Every latch burned and made my whole body tense up. I could tell Lou was feeding well and getting milk, but I was convinced there must be something wrong. With so much preparation and experience supporting others, I was not expecting it to be so uncomfortable. I reached out to my sister, my girlfriends who breastfed, and a lactation consultant, who reminded me that no one had ever sucked on my nipples for hours and hours day and night and that there would be an adjustment period before it got better. One of my girlfriends gave me great advice; she said, "I remember that feeling of dreading the initial latch, but the discomfort should subside shortly after. Try not to let your baby see you wince or hear you cuss in agony. You don't want her to associate breastfeeding with your discomfort. Instead, take a deep breath, smile, and sing a song to distract yourself. By the time you're at the chorus the pain will ease away. You've got this." They were all right. It sucked (no pun intended) for another day, I pushed through, and before I knew it nursing became painless and an absolute joy.

It is important to note that discomfort in the beginning is normal to a certain extent, but it can also be an indication of an issue that needs to be addressed, so please don't neglect asking for help. If painful feeding persists you will want to get support from a friend or lactation consultant as soon as possible to set you on the right path for a successful breastfeeding journey. Sometimes a simple adjustment to a poor latch can make all the difference.

Here are some things that helped me find relief in the early days.

- Use a firm breastfeeding pillow and proper positioning.

- Baby should be tummy to tummy with you so that her head is not turned to the side but instead directly facing your nipple.

- Sandwich your breast to get as much of your areola in baby's mouth.

- Make sure baby's top and bottom lips are flanged out and not rolled inward.

- To help your baby get a nice deep latch, encourage her to open her mouth nice and wide. Rubbing your nipple over her lips or expressing some milk onto her lips encourages baby to open her mouth.

- In between feeds use a silver nursing cup, which has antimicrobial, antifungal, and antibacterial properties.

- Use an organic nipple balm and get fresh air and sunshine without a bra to help soothe and heal.

REPEAT THESE MANTRAS OUT LOUD

I recognize the resilience of my body.
I give thanks for all it has and continues to do for me and my baby.
I am resilient because _____ (fill in the blank).

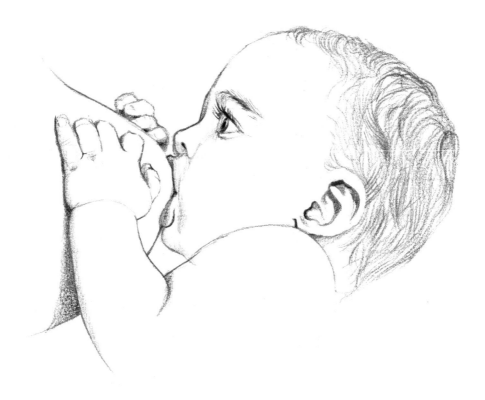

Record Your Birth Story

For this week's activity, I invite you to jot down your birth story. You do not have to spend a lot of time on this journal entry, and you don't have to share it with anyone. For now, just put pen to paper to record the details while they are fresh in your mind.

Once you have finished writing your story, put your pen down and close your eyes. Place one hand over your heart and one hand over your womb space. Take a deep breath into your belly and let it go out of your mouth. Find yourself here exactly where you are without judgment. Briefly scanning your body, take a few more deep breaths into the places of tension of discomfort and exhale completely out of your mouth.

YOUR MAGIC MILK

You made it through your first week of motherhood! Now that your milk has come in and the adrenaline has worn off you may be feeling all the feels as you settle into your new rhythm. In Week 34 I talk about the four pillars of an optimal postpartum period: support, nourishment, rest, and touch. I hope you have set yourself up to be held and mothered through this sacred time. If you're feeling overwhelmed and undersupported, it's never too late to put these pillars in place. I invite you to revisit that week and the corresponding activity to reconnect with your postpartum intentions and community of support.

In your second week you may feel more ease with breastfeeding and like you're getting the hang of it. However, if you are still struggling to find comfort and a good flow, know that your breastfeeding journey is not doomed and that you are not alone in the struggle. The adjustment period that so many new moms experience is often not talked about, but with patience, commitment, and care you can turn a corner. Good things are worth working hard for, and breastfeeding often requires resilience and commitment.

CLOGGED DUCTS AND MASTITIS

Clogged ducts happen when milk is not drained from breastfeeding, causing a blockage in the breast. This may feel like you have a rock stuck in your breast and cause tenderness or a bleb visible from the nipple. When a blocked duct is not cleared it can lead to a breast infection called mastitis. Mastitis is usually accompanied by flulike symptoms (fever, body aches, chills). Although antibiotics are commonly prescribed as treatment for mastitis, they are not always necessary and can lead to unwanted side effects. Here are some tips for managing clogged ducts and mastitis naturally.

Keep Feeding: It is perfectly fine for your baby to continue to feed from the breast with an infection. In fact, it is preferable that they do this to help you clear the blockage. Breastfeed in different positions to encourage milk to flow. Try lying your baby on his back on the bed or floor and dangle your breast over him while on all fours. This is called dangle feeding.

Massage: Use a warm compress to first heat the breast, then use castor oil or another pure carrier oil to gently and firmly massage your breast toward the nipple to encourage drainage. Doing this in the bath or shower can be helpful.

Supplements: Treat mastitis as you would any infection. Minimize sugar, drink lots of water, and take vitamin C, echinacea, zinc, propolis, and probiotics. Sunflower lecithin can help thin your milk and is something to consider if you have reoccurring blockage.

267

Homeopathy: Pulsatilla is useful for helping the milk flow and Belladona can be used for inflammation and fever. Arnica can help with aches and pains.

Salt Soak: Soak your nipple in an Epsom salt solution or take an Epsom salt bath.

To prevent mastitis you want to be sure your baby has a proper latch and is emptying the breast completely with each feed. Ditch restrictive bras or clothing and be mindful not to overstimulate supply.

OPTIMIZING MILK SUPPLY

Breast milk works through supply and demand. The more consistently you nurse, the more milk you make. Here are some other ways to optimize your milk supply.

- Oxytocin triggers milk letdown, so follow the feel-good hormone and spend lots of time skin-to-skin to keep your supply flowing.

- Alternating breasts per feeding or in the middle of a feed is important to help balance out supply.

- Dress your baby in only a diaper to allow for that skin-to-skin contact while feeding.

- Prioritize hydration, good nutrition, and adequate caloric intake. It is crucial that you are getting the proper nutrients and healthy fats you need to produce milk. The postpartum period is not the time to start dieting and calorie restricting. This could put your milk supply at risk.

- Sleeping next to your baby can help make night feedings easier and support oxytocin production. It gives your baby more opportunity to suckle and therefore increase supply.

- Keep stress in check. Healthy stress management and support are important factors for milk supply.

- Include galactagogue (lactation-promoting) foods and herbs in your diet, such as coconut water, oats, ginger, sweet potatoes, fenugreek, shatavari, nettle, red raspberry, spirulina, moringa, and carrots.

- Introducing formula or combo feeding can impact your supply. Formula metabolizes differently and keeps babies full for longer. Therefore, they are more likely to go longer stretches without breastfeeding. The decrease in demand often results in less supply.

Erica's Milk-Rich Seed Bread

This is a recipe from my dear friend Erica Mock, a homesteader in North Carolina whom we get our dairy and meat from. I swore by this gluten-free seed bread to help encourage healthy digestion and milk supply in the first months postpartum.

Makes 2 loaves

1¾ cups [420 ml] water

2 eggs

¼ cup [60 g] melted coconut oil

1 Tbsp maple syrup

2½ cups [250 g] gluten-free rolled oats

½ cup [70 g] raw pumpkin seeds

269

½ cup [70 g] black sesame seeds (freshly ground if desired)

½ cup [80 g] freshly ground flax seeds

½ cup [70 g] almonds

¼ cup [35 g] psyllium husks

2 Tbsp chia seeds

1 tsp fine grain sea salt or ½ tsp coarse salt

Grease two loaf pans with coconut oil.

In a medium bowl, whisk the water, eggs, coconut oil, and maple syrup.

In a large bowl, combine the oats, pumpkin seeds, sesame seeds, flax seeds, almonds, psyllium husks, chia seeds, and salt, stirring well.

Add the wet ingredients to the dry ingredients and mix very well until everything is completely soaked and the dough becomes very thick but manageable.

Scrape the batter into the prepared loaf pans, smooth the top with the back of a spoon, and let sit on the counter for 30 minutes.

Preheat the oven to 350°F [175°C]. Place the loaf pans in the oven on the middle rack and bake for 20 minutes. Remove bread from loaf pans, place them upside down directly on the rack, and bake for another 30 to 40 minutes. The bread is done when it sounds hollow when tapped. Let cool completely before slicing.

To serve, heat in a buttered pan and top with mashed avocado, lemon juice, salt, and sauerkraut.

Store in a tightly sealed container for up to 5 days. The bread also freezes well.

OVERABUNDANCE OF MILK

With so much attention and worry focused on if baby is getting enough milk, many mamas don't realize that having an overabundance of milk can come with challenges too. You may be feeling grateful for your fruitful supply but also wondering how to manage the engorgement and rapid flow. You may find that your flow is so strong that it upsets your baby. The good news is that as hormones level out, your supply will start to balance too. I promise you won't be soaking through your shirt all day and night forever. In the meantime, here are some things to try.

Laid-Back Feeding: Use gravity to slow the flow. Lean back in a reclining position and let your baby feed on top of you.

Pumping and Storing: Although you may need to help your baby empty your breast to prevent any blockage, you'll want to be mindful not to do too much pumping, which will stimulate the breast and signal for more supply. Instead, try using a milk collector that can catch the letdown from the breast you're not feeding with or use it to gently hand express and collect excess. Store this surplus in silicone ice cube trays in the freezer for future use.

Foods to Avoid: Be mindful of consuming galactagogue foods and herbs such as fenugreek, turmeric, or nettle, which could be boosting your supply unknowingly.

TONGUE TIES

There are a lot of conflicting schools of thought about tongue ties, and it is unknown why exactly we are seeing it more in children today. Some speculate it could have to do with folic acid intake; others believe the uptick is because more practitioners are looking for them. If your baby has a lip or tongue tie it can impact breastfeeding, so it is something to look for if you are struggling with latching or breastfeeding. The go-to method of "fixing" a lip or tongue tie is to cut through the tissue. I see this procedure recommended often, even in the absence of breastfeeding challenges.

This procedure can be a useful tool but should not be done without great consideration for the potential side effects, including pain. Although it is considered a minor surgery, it can lead to greater breastfeeding challenges when done unnecessarily or without proper bodywork or rehabilitation. Although my daughter has a very pronounced lip and tongue tie, I chose not to "correct" it because it has not led to any breastfeeding difficulties and the risk of it jeopardizing breastfeeding in the first year is just too great. If you suspect a lip or tongue tie is the cause of your breastfeeding discomfort, get multiple opinions on the best path forward and always utilize the support of a craniosacral and myofascial specialist who can help optimize the function of the tongue with or without the surgical revision.

INTRODUCING A BOTTLE

When, if, and how to introduce a bottle to your baby is a personal choice based on your unique family needs. My general recommendation for breastfeeding mothers is to delay the introduction of a bottle until you and baby feel confident in your breastfeeding rhythm. If a bottle is introduced too early and too often, baby can get accustomed to the steady and easy bottle flow and prefer it to the breast. This can cause babies to resist the breast because they know they must work a bit harder for milk.

Pumping milk and cleaning bottles are extra steps that ultimately make more work for mom, which is why those who breastfeed from the breast tend to breastfeed for longer. Before consistently introducing a bottle, get well acquainted with breastfeeding. If someone else is bottle feeding your baby, it means you are skipping a breastfeed, so you will likely have to pump at the same time to prevent engorgement or supply dip. I much preferred breastfeeding over pumping and sanitizing bottles, and for this reason I never gave Lou a bottle. She eventually learned to drink breast milk from a cup at five months old. Of course, if you have to go back to work outside the home or be apart from your baby in the early months, then a bottle will become necessary and something you will want to practice getting your baby familiar with a week or two prior. Some babies are not big on the bottle right away, but trying different bottle shapes, milk temperatures, and feeding techniques can help them transition.

When you feel ready to start a bottle, opt for a nipple flow that is smaller than recommended for your baby's age. This may mean giving your baby a preemie size nipple. This will allow the milk to flow out more slowly, making the baby work harder at the bottle and more likely to transition from bottle to breast with ease.

273

SWADDLING AND THE STARTLE REFLEX

If you gave birth in the hospital, you were probably taught how to swaddle your baby nice and tight. Nurses swear by swaddling to keep babies feeling snug, safe, and soothed and to prevent them from waking from their startle reflex. You've likely noticed your newborn flinging their arms out to the sides when they hear a loud noise, are placed down, or experience sudden movement. This is a normal and healthy response called the Moro reflex. Swaddling may lead to better sleep for this reason, but what people don't realize is that babies move through and grow out of this reflex not with time but through integration. The more your baby is given the opportunity to move freely through it, the sooner it subsides. Babies don't need swaddles to feel safe and secure; all they need are their mama's loving arms. Swaddle blankets place a barrier between skin-to-skin with mama, which you know by now is incredibly beneficial. Without a swaddle, babies can use their little hands to explore mama's body while feeding. These angelic strokes stimulate oxytocin in mama and promote milk supply. Additionally, when babies are given free range of motion, they are able to use and strengthen their muscles for optimal development. If you choose to swaddle, do so in moderation and make sure your baby is getting plenty of tummy time and skin-to-skin during wake windows.

PACIFIERS AND PACIFYING

When it comes to pacifiers, they can be a helpful resource and if they work for you and your babe, great! What I will say is that I do not recommend introducing a pacifier until a strong milk supply and latch have been well established. When babies cry, they are communicating a need: hunger, connection, closeness, etc. Be mindful not to pacify with a pacifier before meeting the need they are communicating to you. Always offer your baby your breast before a pacifier so you don't miss

274

a feeding cue. My sister once said to me, "I didn't give my kids pacifiers because I didn't want to have to go through the trouble of taking it away from them one day." This resonated with me, so we decided to skip the pacifier too. Some dentists warn against the use of pacifiers because it can have a negative impact on the development and structure of the mouth and teeth, which is something to consider.

A NOTE ON VISITORS

Many new parents feel pressure from loving friends and family eager to come visit and get in on those sweet baby cuddles. In Week 34 I shared that we decided not to have any visitors for three weeks so that we could rest, bond, and integrate into our new routines without feeling like we were hosting others. I didn't feel ready so early on for others to hold Lou and wanted to maximize our skin-to-skin time in those sacred early weeks. In this time, we did, however, have the support of a postpartum doula.

Whenever you feel ready to invite people into your baby bubble is up to you. Don't get caught up in other people's feelings. Your priority is honoring you and your baby's needs and it's okay if that doesn't align with what other people expect from you. If you are accepting visitors, put a sign on the door asking them to remove their shoes, wash their hands, and follow any other requests you may have. Perhaps your guest can help unload the dishwasher while they visit or hold the baby while you take a bath. I always say that during the sacred window all guests need to earn baby cuddles. Have a code word with your partner so that you can politely send away any visitor who is overstaying their welcome.

Your Divine Maternal Purpose

Your baby was born into your family for a reason. Your baby chose you. You are the perfect match for your baby and have within you all that she needs. This human being has come into your life with a divine purpose, and you have been chosen to usher her in and grow alongside her. It is not a coincidence; there is a cosmic consciousness at play. This week, spend some time journaling and reflecting on the gifts you have to offer your child. Meditate on why your child might have chosen you in this lifetime and why she chose to join this family. Acknowledge all the wisdom and love you have to offer and know that all the imperfections are there in service to her too.

GIVE YOURSELF GRACE

The third week of motherhood might feel like you gave birth yesterday and three years ago. It's like running a marathon and a sprint at the same time. The postpartum portal is often described as a place where otherworldly ecstatic bliss and grief come together. It may seem odd to use grief to describe the emotional state that comes with the birth of new life, but parenthood requires us to face the death of our old selves, our old ways of life, our independence. As a result, moving through big emotions is a very normal part of the postpartum experience. Layer on hormone changes and lack of sleep, and some tears are bound to happen! Did you know that the hormonal drop that takes place after birth is the single largest change in hormones in the shortest period of time, including adolescence? If that doesn't put things in perspective, I don't know what will. No matter how grateful you are to be a mom or how deeply in love you are with your baby, this roller coaster of emotions known as the "baby blues" is part of the process for so

277

many and nothing to feel ashamed of. Surround yourself with friends who understand where you're at and who can show up for you without judgment. Give yourself grace as you move through the biggest life transformation one will ever experience.

Lingering or intensified feelings of sadness, helplessness, or debilitating anxiety that persist may suggest a perinatal mood or anxiety disorder. If these feelings become overwhelming or unmanageable and interfere with your ability to care for your baby or experience joy, it's imperative to seek out support as soon as possible.

One in five mothers experience postpartum mood and anxiety disorders (PMADs). The staggering prevalence of PMADs reflects our society's and our economic system's disregard for the needs of new parents. The "mismatch hypothesis" suggests that PMAD rates today are so high because of the radical contrast between modern motherhood and how our ancestors lived.[80] Poor nutrition, limited sun exposure, financial hardship, lack of familial closeness and support, negative birth experience, chronic stress, and early weaning are all risk factors for postpartum depression that so many of us face. Many women mother in isolation or are expected to return to work shortly after birth, creating a great deal of stress, which is why postpartum depression is often referred to as a disease of modern motherhood.[81] I believe the solution depends on a systematic shift that places value on a healthy mother-baby dyad and thriving family above all else.

Pharmaceutical antidepressants specifically formulated and marketed for postpartum depression have emerged on the market over the past few years. The most recent drug lists suicidal thoughts and behavior, sleepiness, and confusion as possible side effects. Patients are instructed not to drive or operate heavy machinery for at least twelve hours after taking the pill, which leaves me wondering how they are expected to safely care for a child. Treatment should always be addressed through a multifaceted approach, looking at potential nutrient deficiencies, thyroid deficiency, hormone imbalances, and lifestyle factors[82] that may be contributing to emotional dysregulation. Therapeutic modalities such as somatic therapy and cognitive behavioral therapy can be very effective.

Below are some evidence-based lifestyle factors you can implement to improve your emotional state and well-being.

- Consider making changes in your professional life to tend to yourself and your child in the season you are in. Honor the hormonal and emotional needs of your baby and body.

- Get more support where it is needed (i.e., therapy, postpartum doula, a support group for new mothers, friends, and family).

- Prioritize balanced blood sugar (see Week 24).

- Get optimal levels of B12, D3, magnesium, copper, and zinc through supplementation and nutrient-rich foods.

- Get your iron levels tested.[83] Consume adequate amounts of iron in your diet, ideally from organ meats (see Week 25).

- Consume adequate protein and fat, especially omega-3s.

- Get at least twenty minutes of sun exposure daily.

- Prioritize social interaction with loved ones.[84]

- Find community of other mothers.

- Exercise daily (even a light walk counts).

- Herbs such as saffron, turmeric, and ashwagandha are all known to alleviate symptoms of depression.

279

A Love Letter to Yourself

One of the biggest myths in our culture is that parents have it all together. This fallacy of perfection plays a huge role in the pressures and unrealistic expectations parents face. The pressure to meet external expectations or even one's own personal expectations can bring up feelings of guilt, shame, and judgment. These feelings keep us from living in the present moment.

Just like a newborn is learning everything for the first time, so are you! You and your baby are growing together. Treating yourself with the same compassion and patience you would your baby is so important. You are resilient. You are capable of feeling the big waves of change and continuing to show up for your baby.

WRITE A LETTER TO YOUR LITTLE ONE SHARING THE JOY AND CHALLENGES YOU FACE

Reveal any insecurities or pressures you may feel on this journey along with the feelings of joy, confidence, excitement, and gratitude. Ask questions. Remind your little one that you too are growing and learning. Let this exercise be a reminder that you, in all your humanness, are everything your baby needs and more. You are strong and capable of riding the waves. It is okay to show your vulnerability and your strength. This letter is just for you.

TAKING MAMA STEPS OUTSIDE THE NEST

By week four you may be feeling ready to step outside your nest a bit or open your home to visitors. Our first car ride with Lou took place at four weeks and it was a bit nerve-racking to leave the nest, but it was a success! In the months following, car rides became a nightmare. She would scream and cry and there was nothing I could do. We would pull over and as soon as she was in my arms and on my breast, she would return to a state of calm. I honestly considered abandoning the car and walking home on the side of the freeway multiple times. I found that sitting in the back seat next to her made things harder, and once she got more acclimated to car rides the solo time in the back led to less tears. What helped her the most (and still does) is kids' music. What did parents do before there was Raffi!?

281

Here is some of the best advice I have gotten when it comes to outings with your babe.

- Opt for a carrier instead of a stroller in the early weeks. You can breastfeed more comfortably in public and having babe close to your chest keeps strangers out of the baby's personal space.

- One of my favorite pieces of advice I got in early motherhood was to always put a hat on my baby in public. Since the baby's fontanel is not fully fused yet, the soft spot on the top of a baby's head allows them a greater connection to the divine. The crown chakra is Sanskrit for "bridge to the cosmos." This opening is symbolic for connection to the spiritual world and head coverings are used across many cultures and religions for energetic protection. Since your baby is highly attuned, a hat acts as a negative energy shield while in public spaces.

- Don't feel the need to cover up when breastfeeding. Do whatever you need to do to be comfortable, but don't worry about making anyone else comfortable while feeding your baby.

BABY WEARING

If I had to choose just one item to purchase for motherhood, it would be a baby carrier. Baby carriers are one of the earliest human inventions and have been in practice for thousands of years across nearly every culture. Benefits include skin-to-skin contact, hands-free baby holding, breastfeeding on the go, contact napping, soothing a fussy baby, and so much more. I have relied on the carrier for writing this book, naps, outings, walks, air travel, and everything in between. Dads love it too!

There are many different carriers to choose from and pros and cons to different styles of baby wearing. Ultimately, it comes down to personal preference and finding the right fit and comfort for your lifestyle. In the newborn period, I loved the soft stretchy fabric of a wrap carrier to wear in the home. As Lou's neck muscles strengthened, the ring sling became a very convenient and stylish way to wear her around the house and on the go. It fit easily in my purse and could come on and off without much fuss. As she grows bigger, I use a structured carrier that allows me to wear her on my front or on my back. This is more supportive for a heavier baby and allows me to take her on long hikes and outings. You don't need to purchase different types for different stages, but if you choose to try a few styles out you can easily resell lightly used ones.

If baby wearing is uncomfortable, make sure you are wearing the carrier correctly. Don't hesitate to reach out to the brand for guidance and tips on troubleshooting. It should not be putting strain on your body. You will also want to follow wearing instructions to be sure your baby's legs are positioned correctly to promote healthy hips.

TIPS FOR A GASSY BABY

Whoever made up the saying "sleeping soundly like a baby" clearly never had a baby. Newborns sleep a lot, but they also wiggle and wake often as gas moves through their newly developed system that is acclimating to digesting milk. It can be unsettling to see your baby uncomfortable, but know that for the most part a gassy baby who finds relief once gas has passed is normal and will improve with time.

Try holding your baby upright with his knees bent up to his belly in a squat position.

Bicycle baby's legs while he is on his back or give him a gentle belly massage with oil.

283

A warm bath can help relax the stomach muscles and soothe the nervous system.

Sometimes mama's diet can have an impact, so if you suspect that there could be a correlation you can try removing dairy, brassicas, spicy foods, raw foods, or caffeine from your diet (one at a time). These tend to be the most common culprits, although every baby is unique.

PARENTING IN THE AGE OF AI

Today there are hundreds of apps, gadgets and hi-tech baby monitors marketed to new parents to keep track of feeds, wakes, poops, and pees and promising to "make motherhood easier." Frankly I'm exhausted just thinking about it. I can say with confidence, these inventions do not make motherhood easier. They do not help us parent better nor do they alleviate anxiety. Instead, they take us further from the present moment, our intuition, and make us more reliant on the devices that are intruding more and more into our daily lives. The baby monitors that detect breathing patterns, REM cycles, wet diapers, temperature, track movement, and literally rock your baby really aren't that impressive to me. We as parents have been successfully doing all these things for centuries. They are a bandage approach in a world that is disconnected to nurture, community, and emotional well-being.

What if I told you that you and your baby could thrive without a schedule or a performance review from an app? What if I told you that you are fully capable of tuning into your child's rhythms and meeting her needs, without living under the shadow of Big Tech?

Use your hand to feel the temperature of her skin, smell her diaper to know if it's clean, let her chest rise and fall on your body as she sleeps, offer your breast to her when she cries and you'll know if she's hungry. You see, nature has provided us with the tools we need to tune in. Using our senses strengthens our trust in ourselves and our children.

5 x 5 x 7
Breathwork for Stability & Centeredness

This can be done anytime you need a nervous system reset, such as while you are cooking, driving, or playing with your child, or when your child is upset and needs to co-regulate with you. Slowing your breath signals to your brain and nervous system that you are safe.

Relax your eyebrows, the area around your eyes, and your tongue and unclench your jaw. Roll your shoulders forward five times and then roll them backward five times. Inhale for 5 seconds through your nose, hold your breath for 5 seconds, and slowly exhale for 7 seconds. Whenever you are ready, continue this for five cycles: Inhale through your nose for 5, hold for 5, exhale for 7.

As you are inhaling, imagine your breath as a healing force that is slowing down your heart rate. Visualize your heart rate on a speedometer and as you inhale, the speedometer slowly begins to decelerate, as your "engine" slows down. Every inhale you take, you are slowing down your heart rate; with every exhale, you are pushing deeper into your source of stability and centeredness.

NUTRIENTS TO CONSIDER IN THE FOURTH TRIMESTER

During pregnancy there is so much emphasis on nourishing mothers to support fetal development, but once baby is born many women focus their attention on baby and forget that supplementation and optimal nutrients after birth are just as important for replenishing their reserves and enriching breast milk. Babies continue to benefit from their mother's nutrients long after birth, which is why it is recommended to continue to take your prenatal supplements throughout the duration of breastfeeding. The postpartum period is not the time to restrict calories or try to fit back into your old jeans. It is a time when we need even more nourishment to restore our bodies and feed our growing babies. You will want to maintain focus on saturated fats, proteins, complete carbohydrates, iron-rich foods, choline, and omega-3s for brain health; calcium for all the milk you are producing; and vitamin C to help synthesize collagen for skin and hair growth.

In addition to the vitamins and minerals listed in Weeks 4, 14, and 25, here are three additional nutrients of particular importance in the fourth trimester.

Iodine: Iodine is a mineral that is essential for healthy thyroid, brain, and nervous system function. Iodine benefits baby's brain development and thyroid function too and is reliant on mom's stores in breast milk to attain optimal levels. • **Where to find it:** *Seafood, seaweed, poultry, liver, beef, egg, dairy, beans*

Selenium: This mineral works in conjunction with iodine to maintain healthy thyroid function. It has been shown to significantly decrease the incidence of postpartum thyroiditis. Optimal levels may be protective against postpartum depression. It is also known to help maintain healthy hair growth. We will talk more about postpartum hair loss and growth in Week 9 Earthside. • **Where to find it:** *Brazil nuts, seafood, organ meats, eggs*

Ashwagandha: This adaptogen has been used medicinally for hundreds of years. It is beneficial in helping alleviate stress, anxiety, inflammation, and fatigue. It boosts energy, immune system function, and libido. This herb is a wonderful resource for new mamas who are in need of some extra support as they navigate less sleep and new rhythms.

Lymphatic Breast Massage

WITH LISA LEVITT GAINSLEY

I first met Lisa Levitt Gainsley, author of *The Book of Lymph*, when I began working as a doula. I heard through the grapevine about her magic touch, deep wisdom, and experience as a certified lymphedema therapist. When I booked an appointment to see her she looked at my intake form and said, "Is your grandmother Edith?" Turns out she had supported my grandmother, who had passed away nearly fifteen years prior, while she underwent chemotherapy. Needless to say, it was a full circle moment that made her work even more special to me. Lisa has played an important role in the healing of so many people in our community.

Breast self-massage can help reduce inflammation, ease engorgement, flush out excess waste in the tissues, boost your immune system, and help maintain fluid balance. Your lymphatic system is the great recycling system of your body, circulating immune cells and clearing out excess bacteria, toxins, hormones, and even fat in your gut. Your lymph system depends on muscle contractions, pulsing of arteries, exercise, deep breathing, and lymphatic massage to move lymph fluid. That's why giving yourself a lymphatic massage can help alleviate congestion in your body.

Wait a few weeks after birth before starting lymphatic massage, giving your body time to adjust and your milk to come in. Lymphatic breast self-massage can help mitigate some of the fullness you may be feeling.

You can soften the landscape of your breasts with a gentle, nurturing touch. Become intimate with the changes of your breasts and the terrain of your breast tissue. Cultivate loving-kindness and recognize that when you are massaging your breasts, you are improving lymphatic circulation to help clear stagnation and create a more harmonious landscape as well as maintaining breast health.

Below is a breast self-massage sequence to support lactation and help stave off mastitis, breast pain, and clogged milk ducts. Please note: Do not work on yourself when you have an active, acute infection.

BEFORE YOU BEGIN

Please follow these simple massage principles:

- **Understand the lymphatic drainage pattern of your breasts.** You will massage the main lymph nodes at your neck first. These lymph nodes move fluid back to your bloodstream. The lymph fluid from your breasts drains to the axillary nodes in your armpits and along the center of your chest. Always stimulate these nodes before massaging your breasts.

- **Use an extra-light touch.** Lymphatic massage is gentle. You're working the fluid layer above the muscle bed. Your strokes should be soft and nurturing, just like how you would soothe your baby. It will also calm your nervous system and allow you to enter the rest and digest state.

- **Work slowly.** Your lymph system moves six to twelve times per minute. Stay in this rhythm. You only need to work for a few minutes. You don't need to detoxify your body too quickly.

- **Use skin-on-skin contact for maximum benefit.**

- **Massage your breasts after you've breastfed your baby or pumped.**

- **Drink plenty of water afterward.**

STEP-BY-STEP SELF-CARE ROUTINE

You can do this a few times a week. I hope you enjoy it!

1 **Massage the lymph nodes at the base of your neck.** The supraclavicular lymph nodes are just above your collarbone. Gently press your fingertips down into the hollows above your collarbone, making a J motion down and out toward your shoulders. Repeat ten times.

2 **Stimulate the axillary lymph nodes in your armpits.** There are three steps:

   01 Place your hand inside your armpit. Pulse upward into your armpit. Repeat ten times.

   02 Place your hand a little farther down the side of your torso. This region contains breast tissue, which is essential to drain. With the palm of your hand, make C strokes up the side of your torso into your armpit. Repeat ten times.

   03 Lift your arm and place your hand into your armpit. Pump over your armpit ten times.

3 **Massage the tops of your shoulders**. I call this your shirt-collar lymphatic zone. Place your hands on top of your shoulders, your elbows pointing straight in front of you. Inhale, then drop your elbows as you exhale, keeping your fingertips on your shoulders. This helps move lymphatic fluid from the back of your neck to the nodes above your collarbone and is fantastic for releasing neck tension. Repeat five times.

4 **Stretch your neck.** Drop your right ear to your right shoulder. Hold for three seconds, breathing in and out deeply. Then drop your left ear to your left shoulder. Hold and breathe. Repeat two times. If you're comfortable you can make small circles with your head in both directions. Stretching your neck will reduce muscle tension from breastfeeding that may be impeding lymph flow.

5 **Draw rainbows over your chest, which is great for calming worry and anxiety.** Place the palm of one hand in the center of your chest, over your breastbone. Take a slow, deep breath and feel your chest rise into your hand. Exhale slowly, feeling your chest relax. Take another breath in and feel your chest rise into your hand. As you exhale, feel your chest relax. Massage upside-down C strokes over your heart and lungs. This is where your heart chakra lies; treat it with acceptance, self-love, and tenderness. Repeat ten times.

6 **Massage the top of your breast.** Place the palm of your hand above your breast, your fingertips facing your armpit. Gently massage C strokes over the top of your breast toward your armpit. Repeat five times.

7 **Massage the axillary lymph nodes in your armpit again five times.**

8 **Massage your breast under the bra line.** Place your palm underneath your breast. Gently, like a wave, massage C strokes toward the side of your torso, then up into your armpit. Repeat three times.

9 **Lightly tap your sternum.** Visualize the sound of the thumping down into your cells. This is where the thymus is located, above your heart. The thymus stores white blood cells that become active T cells when they need to mount an immune response.

10   **Repeat step 6,** massaging the top of your breast toward your armpit.

11   **Gently knead your entire breast.** Massage the fluid away from your nipple. Think of the sun's rays radiating from the nipple outward. Some of the fluid in your breast will drain into the lymph nodes along your sternum, called the internal chain of mammary lymph nodes, as well as the axillary lymph nodes in your armpit. Notice how your breasts feel. They may be tender or full. Focus your thoughts and attention on softening the area. Create a nurturing environment here. I often say that the more time you take to get to know your body, the more you are cultivating a new landscape.

12   **Repeat step 8,** massaging your breast under the bra line.

13   **Repeat step 2,** stimulating the axillary lymph nodes in your armpit.

14   **Repeat step 3,** stimulating your shirt-collar lymphatic zone.

15   **Repeat step 1,** stimulating the right and left supraclavicular lymphatic nodes at the base of your neck.

16   **Repeat steps 2 to 12 on your other breast.**

NOTE

If you've had breast cancer, a lumpectomy, lymph node removal, surgery, reconstruction, radiation, or biopsies, please consult your physician or a certified lymphedema therapist for clearance. If you've had a breast reduction, lift, or augmentation, the gentle techniques of lymphatic massage are beneficial for healing trauma in the tissues.

For more information, please refer to Lisa's book, *The Book of Lymph*, available wherever books are sold.

CLOSING THE PORTAL

This week is considered the end of the postpartum period according to Western medicine. At six weeks women will see their obstetricians for the first and last time after birth. This short visit may include a prescription for birth control pills and the clearance to have sex again. This appointment is often described as completely void of the support one actually desires and is reflective of our culture and health care system's failure to meet the needs of postpartum mothers. This six-week mark does not mean that from one day to the next you are no longer postpartum or that you should feel completely healed physically or emotionally, as healing is not linear. For those honoring the Eastern practice of "sitting in" and resting for the first forty days, this week is also symbolic of the end of one chapter and the beginning of the next phase of matrescence. You are moving through one portal to the next.

Knowing the importance of the first forty days postpartum on maternal and infant health, I gave myself a lot of grace in those six

294

weeks. I took all the time and rest I needed and I embraced my wide hips and soft belly with amazement and admiration. When that six-week/forty-day postpartum mark approached, I could feel the pressure to "bounce back" bubble up within me. Even though I knew there was no such thing as a universal end date to the postpartum period nor would there ever be a return to my old self, my old body, or my old life, somewhere within me I was holding on to the belief that at six weeks I would feel complete. Six weeks came and went but my clothes still didn't fit, I was not ready to have sex, and my vagina still felt foreign and daunting to even look at.

I texted my midwife, feeling defeated and like something was wrong with me. She reminded me to be patient and that with time and gentle movement I would rediscover a connection with my body. She was right. What helped tremendously was a session with a pelvic floor therapist who gave me specific feedback on where I was holding tension and where I could work on strengthening. She also gave me some exercises to do. (Refer back to Week 15 for more info on pelvic floor.) Reconnecting with my pelvic floor in this way made me feel more ready to be physically and sexually active again. Honor where your body is at before jumping back into your old routines. Take it slow and expect it to feel different for a while. If pain presents, take a step back and seek support from a pelvic health specialist. The yoga sequence in Week 25 can be used to gently introduce movement in the postpartum period too.

This week is a time of integration for the physical and emotional body. In Mexican traditions, midwives perform a "closing of the bones" ceremony, which utilizes massage, herbal steaming, bathing, and swaddling the new mother in a sacred tapestry called the rebozo. The wrapping that takes place creates a firm embrace around the hips and womb space that have opened physically and energetically. This ritual signifies the closure of the postpartum portal and integration of motherhood.

Postpartum Check-In

Since true postpartum care and attention are lacking within the health care system, I came up with a list of questions for you to use to assess your healing and integration post birth physically and emotionally. Use this as a road map to see where you could use more support and nourishment.

MIND AND BODY

- How is your overall emotional state?

- When do you feel the most overwhelmed?

- Do you feel more anxious than usual?

- What helps you feel your best?

- What self-care rituals have you been prioritizing?

- How much time are you spending on social media?
  How does it make you feel?

- Do you have a supportive community of other mothers to turn to?

- What physical sensations do you feel in your body?

- How are you nourishing yourself?

- Are you eating at least three meals a day with a balance of
  healthy fat, protein, and complete carbohydrates?

- Where can you add more protein into your diet?

- Are you taking any supplements?

- How are you sleeping at night?

- Have you been incorporating gentle movement such as walking
  or stretching? If not, do you feel ready to do so?

- Do you have a meditation or spiritual practice that helps
  ground you?

- Do you feel well supported by your family and friends?

BREASTFEEDING

- How is breastfeeding going? Are you needing any support or encouragement to help you mentally and physically continue breastfeeding?

RELATIONSHIP

- How are you and your partner navigating conflict? How might you both be able to improve communication?
- Are you feeling physically ready to be sexually active?
- Are you feeling emotionally ready to be sexually active?
- Has your cycle returned? If so, are you tracking and taking inventory of your symptoms?
- Have you talked to your partner about how you both plan to prevent pregnancy until you are ready to have another baby?

WORK LIFE

- If you plan to return to work, how are you feeling about it?
- Have your professional goals changed since giving birth?
- How might you be able to honor those changes to support you in the season you are in?

INTEGRATING YOUR BIRTH STORY

with Dr. Maura Moynihan

This week my dear friend Dr. Maura Moynihan is going to guide you through an exercise to help you process your birth story somatically. Dr. Maura specializes in energy medicine, chiropractic, and breathwork and holds a PhD in spiritual psychology. We met in North Carolina after both moving from California around the same time. It felt like a gift from the universe to make a new friend with so much personal and professional mama wisdom. Did I mention she has four teenage boys? Throughout my pregnancy I received bodywork from her and she helped me recognize that we all have the power to transmute any negative state into a rich experience. Every obstacle is a gift inviting us to deepen our connection to ourselves and our life purpose. This is

299

an activity for everyone to partake in but speaks directly to those who are seeking guidance to heal from a traumatic birth experience:

Your birth is designed to teach you how to mother, to strengthen the qualities and attributes your next chapter holds. It's designed to break you out of the illusion of control and soften into the expanse of the intelligence of nature.

After months or even years of dreaming and preparing for your ideal vision for your birth, having spent time and energy on your birth intentions, support system, and the physical and emotional preparation, the birth process ultimately calls for surrender. There are only a handful of times in life when we meet ourselves with such vulnerability, and it is so natural and normal for feelings of shame, despair, guilt, or even rage to come up when our desire to open and birth the way we want does not go to plan. Sometimes our births unfold picture perfect, yet we still have these feelings. Without a spiritual context and support of a community of elders who have gone through this portal and all its iterations, it is natural for us to blame ourselves, our body, our will, our voice, our team, or the circumstances. It is natural to blame because it is just so painful to accept the way things unfolded.

All artists know that the process of inspiration into a final product is a process of unraveling and breaking apart even more than it is the process of coming together. All creation happens this way. When things go wildly off plan, all the emotions that come up are a part of the portal. This means that everything that comes up inside is an energetic wisdom meant to be felt all the way through. It is how we birth ourselves.

What is very important in this process is to have a compassionate ear to hear and hold you as the feelings wash over you. If you do not have someone who can hold a loving space for you without giving advice, thinking that your process should be on a certain timeline or look a certain way, that's okay, because ultimately it comes down to you being with you.

The most important piece is to understand that Life is kind and intelligent. You are an expression of Life. Your baby is an expression of Life. You will continue to be taught and shown your path, and that will be far and away greater than what your mind can understand. When there are turns in the road, Life is preparing us for a greater perspective of Life's unfolding.

Inner Experiencing for Outer Expansion

WITH DR. MAURA MOYNIHAN

1 **Recognize that your feelings are the energetic blueprint for your wholeness and well-being.** Your emotions (energy in motion) when felt all the way through carry the wisdom of healing.

2 **Lie down and get comfortable, and be sure to create a quiet space where you will not be disturbed.** Relax and invite your body, part by part, to rest on the ground. Imagine the Great Mother catching you and embracing your body as you soften into her.

3 **Take a scan of your body for any areas that feel activated or hold sensation.** The body communicates with sensation, so all we need to do is turn toward it for her guidance.

4 **The health of the body is expressed through the energy that flows.** When we can simply feel the sensation that our body holds without getting into a story about it, the energy moves through our meridians in about ninety seconds. This is based in Buddhism and has later been proven with neuroscience. When we can simply feel the energy in our body and allow it, it will surge like a wave and then taper. After the taper an insight will come. It will take as many times as it will take for the waves to move through, and as you do this, the intensity will decrease more and more and the deep well of mothering wisdom will bubble up and show you the very next step to take.

5   **While focusing on the sensation, check to see whether it has a temperature or a texture.** Breathe into the area and ground yourself. Does the sensation have a color? Hold a memory? Does it have a word or a name? Keep your curiosity on the sensation. What quality does it have? Is it sharp, dull, achy, throbby, etc.? Take your time; the mind speeds things up, but the body does not rush. Is there an emotion there? If so, explore what it feels like. See how the body responds to feeling it.

6   **When the sensation releases, place your hand on that part of your body.** Breathe into that area and feel your life force flowing in and out. As the Great Mother holds you, imagine her lovingly giving you whatever it is that you desire. You can receive as much as you want, because her supply is infinite and loving.

Return to this process as much as you need. I have had mothers who do this every day for thirty-three days. What they tend to notice is that after the first few sessions, the process becomes less emotional and more relaxing. There is no right way to do this; it's simply meeting yourself wherever you are and greeting your needs with love.

YOU ARE MOTHERING YOURSELF.

INFANT POTTY LEARNING

A few years ago, I went over to a client's house to visit her and her new baby. As we were talking, her newborn made a sound and my client pulled out what looked like an upside-down plastic top hat, undressed her baby, and positioned her over it while making a "pssssss" noise. *What is she doing?* I thought to myself. She explained to me that she was practicing infant potty learning, otherwise known as elimination communication. Although I was impressed, I was skeptical. I had never before come across this approach, and I was convinced it was only for the crunchiest of moms who had a lot of extra time on their hands to clean up accidents all over the floor.

Years later when Lou was a few weeks old her pediatrician asked me if I was familiar with elimination communication (EC). "Yeah, no thanks. I have enough on my plate," I answered. She assured me that if we started EC it didn't mean having to go without a diaper. I could start at my own pace and just incorporate the potty when I wanted to. It didn't have to be all or nothing. She suggested I begin by making sound associations like "pssss" when I saw her peeing and a grunt sound when I noticed her pooping. Once I started to catch on to her potty cues I would simply bring her to her potty, remove her diaper, and place her on it while providing positive reinforcement with the corresponding sounds. After my pediatrician told me that her daughter was completely diaper free at eighteen months old, I decided to give it a try. At two months we introduced the potty, and I must admit it's become one of the most fun and rewarding practices of parenthood. Our daughter, who couldn't even sit up on her own yet, caught on instantly and displayed a sense of pride whenever she used her potty.

It soon made perfect sense why they call it elimination communication. There was no training involved. It is all based around observation and communication. It's my job to listen for her cues and then respond accordingly. Babies communicate to us all day long, and this was no different. As funny as it may sound, I felt our bond grow even stronger in the weeks that followed. I had been wildly underestimating what she was capable of and how profoundly intelligent the infant brain is.

The benefits aren't just fewer messy blowouts, tushy rashes, skipping potty training, and less dollars spent on diapers. This method is beneficial for a baby's self-esteem and body awareness. We can all relate to wanting to be heard and wanting to stay dry. It turns out that before the "diaper industry" became a thing, early potty learning was actually the norm. It comes as no surprise to learn that pediatricians were incentivized and studies were paid for by leading diaper manufacturers to encourage longer use of diapers than historically appropriate. Pull-ups are a relatively new concept, as are disposable diapers, which have only been around for less than a century!

For us, EC is not goal-oriented potty "training" or an effort to ditch diapers completely. She wears a diaper most of the day and all night.

305

There are many times when I miss her cues (especially pee!). However, I am hopeful that when it comes time for her to be diaper free she will be more familiar with her potty and we will all become more attuned in the meantime.

Respectful Communication

If EC sounds like something you want to practice, give it a try! Whether or not this approach resonates with you, there are many different ways you can strengthen your communication with your baby to better understand her needs and model respectful communication.

When you change your baby's diaper, take her in and out of the car seat, pick her up or put her down, you pass your baby to someone, or bring her to a new place, explain to your baby what to expect and what you are doing. "I am going to change your diaper now," "I am wiping your vagina so that you are all clean," "The doctor is going to use her instrument to examine the inside of your ears."

Something I have observed from mindful bodyworkers, practitioners, and care providers is that they will always communicate to the baby directly, respecting their bodily autonomy and acknowledging their humanness just as one would when engaging with an adult. As you communicate with your baby, notice how she communicates back to you. The more you tune in and observe your baby's cues, the more you will start to be able to distinguish between the different sounds, facial expressions, and movements. Babies are born with the innate ability to communicate. I also believe this practice can be beneficial in nurturing your child's language development skills.

HAIR CARE

Around two months postpartum some mamas start to see the dreaded chunks of hair in their brush, shower, and, well, all over the house! Postpartum shedding can start immediately or go unnoticed until it peaks around four months after birth. No matter how many times people tell you that it is common and temporary, it is still startling to experience it for yourself. A certain amount of postpartum hair loss is to be expected and should not be any cause for concern. Pregnancy hormone shifts change your hair growth cycle, which is why those pregnancy locks are so luscious! When estrogen and progesterone levels shift postpartum, the hair you gained in pregnancy may start to shed, leading to the appearance of more loss than usual. Some extra shedding is not a cause for concern, but excessive or prolonged hair loss can be a sign of mineral deficiency, thyroid dysfunction, or hormone imbalance. The body is always showing us what we need to better our health. If you are losing a lot of hair, don't panic; instead, thank your body for demanding your attention and showing you that it too deserves that TLC.

Although postpartum alopecia is understudied, there are lifestyle choices that can be made to strengthen your hair and provide more fullness. Research on sheep has found greater postpartum hair loss with higher levels of prolactin and cortisol, and lower levels of zinc, copper, and calcium.[85] The correlation between hormones, stress, nutritional deficiencies, and postpartum hair loss tells us that we can take an active approach in prevention. Here are some things to consider.

Thyroid Panel: Work with an integrative or functional medicine doctor to get an in-depth blood panel that looks at your vitamins, minerals, and a full thyroid panel that checks your TSH, T4 ,T3 uptake, total T3, free T4, free T3, reverse T3, and thyroid antibodies. Many deficiencies and markers get overlooked by conventional labs that only test for TSH and T4.

Biotin: Biotin deficiency is known to cause hair loss. Improving levels can greatly increase hair growth.

Silica: This mineral is effective for promoting regrowth by stimulating blood circulation at the scalp and helps with collagen formation.

Collagen: Collagen is an essential protein for healthy skin, nails, connective tissue, and hair. Breastfeeding requires greater protein intake and you will find collagen in protein-rich animal foods.

Nutrient-Rich Diet: Ensure you are eating a sufficient amount of healthy fats, omega-3s, and iron-rich foods.

Pearl Powder: Nacre is a natural compound in pearl powder that stimulates collagen to regenerate. It is also a source of calcium, which can be depleted through pregnancy and breastfeeding. It is rich in silica and other trace minerals.

Stress Management: Hormone health and stress go hand in hand. Finding ways to manage stress will ultimately lead to healthy hair. Consistent exercise is a surefire way to keep stress in check. Apoptogenic herbs may help too.

Hair Hydration: Through pregnancy and the postpartum period I relied heavily on the C & The Moon Glow Oil I formulated. This organic topical hair oil contains jojoba and argan oil, which have both been used for centuries to deliver healthy, gorgeous locks.

Nettles Infusion: A daily nettle infusion can provide minerals to support your adrenals. In a mason jar, steep 2 Tbsp organic dried nettle leaf in 2 cups [480 ml] boiling water for 1 hour.

Shedding the Old to Make Way for the New

Motherhood asks us to shed more than hair strands. It also requires us to shed old parts of ourselves to make way for the new. Spend some time journaling about the parts of yourself that need to be shed for more ease in motherhood. What elements are no longer serving you? What aspects of your old self can you let go of to create more emotional space for the chapter you are in?

BABY SLEEP AND FAMILY PROGRESSIONS

Your baby is waking up to the world more and more each day. Before becoming a mom myself I did not realize how short the sleepy newborn stage is. I thought I would have a little newborn asleep on my chest all day . . . forever. Although it has been magic to watch my daughter's curiosity bloom and her development accelerate before my eyes, I was not prepared for wake windows, playtime, and an overtired baby so early on. I soon learned that each developmental leap comes with growing pains for the entire family. You may be familiar with the term "sleep regression," which is often used to describe these upheavals in a baby's rhythm as they meet new developmental milestones. Regression has a negative connotation, so I find it helpful to call them family progressions as a little reminder that when things get tough, you're growing stronger and more resilient together.

A few weeks ago I was visiting my best friend and her new baby, who is five weeks old. She asked me, "So when does it get easier?" "Who told you it gets easier?" I said. We laughed a little and cried a little and I told her that so many aspects will get easier in time and simultaneously so many new challenges will arise. Just when you think you have it all figured out . . . a new season will arrive to shake things up and keep you on your toes. The ebbs and flows of parenthood are a lot like labor. It looks different for all of us but takes each of us to the point where we have no choice but to become even stronger than we ever thought possible, to expand our hearts and our capacity to unimaginable heights. We ride the waves time and time again. Sometimes we get sucked into the whitewash, but we come out the other side with more courage and better equipped to carry on. There is no feeling more rewarding.

One area that can be the most stressful for new parents is sleep. There is so much external pressure and expectation around infant sleep. Should my baby sleep through the night? Should I train my baby to sleep alone? Should I put my baby on a schedule? The "shoulds" and "should nots" are endless and everyone seems to have the answer. I am no expert in infant sleep, but what if I told you that you don't need an expert? In fact, the only expert on your baby is YOU!

Every so often on a tired day I find myself falling into the trap of thinking I did something wrong. I spiral into late-night Google searches and impulse purchases marketed toward tired moms. Baby sleep is big business! We've been sold lies that babies need to be trained how to sleep, that with proper training they can and should sleep through the night, and that we need to impose hard boundaries on infants to prevent bad habits from forming. These lies have set parents up for failure and placed inappropriate expectations on newborns. Regimented sleep training and the "cry it out" methods are designed to fill the gap of lack of support parents have in a modern world and come at the expense of our children.

313

Every mother's innate instinct is to respond to the cries of her baby. Please don't let anyone convince you that by doing this you are doing anything wrong. Responding to your baby's cries provides them a secure foundation that will serve them their entire life. Your baby's need for connection and closeness is no less important when the sun goes down, and there is no such thing as a "self-soothing" infant. Babies rely on our nervous system to co-regulate and when we respond to their cries it reinforces a feeling of safety that is crucial to their neurological development. Some babies are inherently "good" sleepers, but a waking baby is also a healthy baby who knows that greater arousal prevents SIDS, boosts your milk supply, and helps them get the calories they need to grow.

The days where I get stuck in the idea of how it "should" look are hands down the hardest days for all of us. When I am reminded that it's all part of the process and won't last forever, when I surrender to the ebb and flow and let go of expectations around how and when sleep should happen, we all feel more rested and at ease. It always helps to come back to the reality that the only constant in parenthood is change.

Something I want to emphasize, and I know this to be true from personal experience, is if you rely on your child's naps or bedtime to get work and chores done, have time to yourself, or fulfill basic needs like showering or eating, then you will resent your child for not napping at the time and for the length you want them to. Carve out the support you need from your partner, family, friends, or a hired care provider to take pressure off of both you and your baby around sleep.

Turn to Week 32 to revisit my chapter on co-sleeping, which can also be a helpful sleep solution for many families.

The Rooted Anchor

Close your eyes and visualize a boat floating in the middle of the ocean. From the bottom of the boat a long chain falls to the ocean floor, where it is attached to a big strong anchor. As a storm passes through and the water starts to swell and waves crash onto the boat in chaos, the anchor at the bottom of the sea is still and steady.

As mothers, we are no strangers to the storm. When your child's big emotions sweep in like a force of nature, visualize your boat swaying on top of the sea and the anchor that signifies your stability and calmness. From this place, you can meet your child in the moment, holding space for their need to express big emotions without losing control of yours.

ACCEPTING CHANGE

As much as I wanted to, I knew I couldn't stay in bed cuddling my baby forever and that I had a business to return to and clients to tend to. I had done an excellent job setting myself up for the most supported and relaxing maternity leave, but that time had come to an end and a new chapter was here, one I felt far less prepared for. How was I going to integrate into my new life as a working mother while also finding time to tend to myself? My friendships? My work? Writing a book had long been a dream of mine. The opportunity presented itself in a time of great inspiration and an era where I was straddling two worlds and navigating my new role as a mother.

Writing this book, consulting with clients virtually, hosting circles, and running my skin care line C & The Moon affords me the luxury of working from home. Both Johnathan and I work from home and in the first year of Lou's life she has always been in the presence of either myself or her father. It may sound crazy to some people that we haven't

316

been on a solo date night or left her alone with a caretaker for a whole year. That time will eventually come, but for now it is a privilege we do not take for granted to be able to be near her, and both partake in the daily caretaking role, in this pivotal time of development. Truth be told, there is nowhere we would rather be. This closeness allows me to breastfeed her throughout the day as needed and nurse her to sleep for naps and to look after her alongside a loving hired caretaker. I share this not because I believe it is the right way for all, nor is it possible for everyone, but in hopes to demonstrate that parenthood will inevitably change your usual routine, and that doesn't have to be a bad thing.

The notion that we must leave the home to reclaim ourselves or have space from our children to connect with our greater purpose is a very modern concept that doesn't serve everyone. Motherhood changes you, your identity, your priorities, your friendships, your relationships, your ambitions, and your professional life. For some, having a career fills their cups, allowing them to show up to motherhood with greater energy and presence; for others, work can be draining and a battle against a desire to be home with your child. In our economic paradigm, not going back to work may not be an option. In 2023 it was reported that the average worker spends 27 percent of their income on childcare for children under five.[86] These astronomical costs may require you to reevaluate your current work situation.

The generation before us was set on the belief that women can and should have it all: the independence, financial success, a happy family, a place in the workforce to be of real "value" or to be an "empowered" woman. Being a mother is the most profound contribution one can ever make in the world. Never forget that. If you feel called to spend this season with mothering as your sole focus, do so with pride. If you are a working mama, acknowledge that you too are being in service to your family and release any guilt that keeps you from being present in

317

either role. Check in with yourself and how motherhood has shifted your priorities. Tune out the external expectations or cultural conditioning you may have been sold and follow the path that serves you. There is no formula; the only right way is the one that resonates with you and the unique needs of your family.

Whether you are a stay-at-home mom, work from home, or have a job outside the home, you will need to lean on others. Stay-at-home parenting is not a full-time job; it is a 24/7 job and deserves recognition, respect, and healthy boundaries to avoid burnout. Having community, family support, or hired help is essential for your sanity and ability to fulfill your roles and fill up your cup.

RETURNING TO WORK

If you are returning to work or going to be away from your baby, here are some tips that can help with a smooth transition.

- Talk to your baby and prepare him or her for any change in routine that will come. Explain to your baby where you will be going and why. Assure your baby that he or she will be well cared for while you are gone and that you will be back.

- Plan to have childcare start at least a week before you return to work. Spend time all together so that you and your baby have time to become comfortable and connected before you leave the house. This also allows the caretaker to observe how you mother and learn from your unique approach. If you feel comfortable and safe around this person, it will help your baby feel the same.

- Ask this person to refrain from wearing harsh fragrances and scented laundry detergent in the home. Not only do most

318

fragrances contain endocrine-disrupting chemicals, but babies rely on familiar scent for comfort.

- Invisible String: My mom used to read me a book called *The Invisible String* that taught about the heart connection that cannot be seen but felt near and far. This children's book is equally, if not more, valuable for parents struggling with separation.

- Many working mamas are extra passionate about co-sleeping. The cuddles and connection that take place through the night can help make up for time spent apart during the day. See Week 32 for more on co-sleeping.

319

Taking Temporary Pause

Early motherhood asks a lot of us and that is by design. Our babies need us, but they won't forever. What is one thing you can take off your plate to allow for greater balance and harmony in your life right now? This doesn't have to be a permanent release but can be a temporary pause from an aspect of your life that is causing strain on your ability to mother with ease. What might this look like for you?

PERSPECTIVE IS EVERYTHING

"You'll never sleep again," "Say goodbye to your freedom," "Isn't it exhausting?" People are so quick to impose doom and gloom on new parents, but I'll never forget the ones who said things like "Cherish every moment, it's life's greatest season," or "Just you wait, every day is even sweeter than the next." These people unknowingly taught me the most valuable lesson of parenthood: you get to co-create the experience you want to have and the energy that surrounds your family. Perspective is a choice. Perspective is everything.

Don't get me wrong. Some days are really hard and the best remedy is calling up a girlfriend and having a good old-fashioned vent. When we share our challenges, we feel less alone. This isn't about suppressing our feelings or portraying a false image of perfection. What I am inviting you to do is to reframe the narrative. No matter what your circumstances are, no matter how hard things are at any given moment, the one factor you can control is your outlook. When we choose to see ourselves

321

as victims of this experience, then our perception becomes reality. What if we were to normalize motherhood as an absolute privilege and the greatest spiritual act of service? What if we were to recognize our strength and resilience and commit ourselves fully to mothering from a place of joy and harmony, giving ourselves fully to the experience?

A NOTE ON RESILIENCE

Phil Stutz, a psychiatrist who has helped me through big life challenges, writes, "Inner strength comes only to those who move forward in the face of adversity. We're trained as a society to expect, even demand, immediate gratification. And we have an extraordinary ability to rationalize this weakness."[87]

We are living in a time where mental health struggles are becoming destigmatized, self-care is celebrated, and the value of rest is finally recognized. With this important paradigm shift it is easy to forget that there is great wisdom and value in the uncomfortable when we learn to embrace it.

If you've made it this far in the book, you know that I am deeply passionate about mothers feeling held and supported in every way. After all, that's what this book is about. However, I often hear people say, "You should just stop breastfeeding if it's taking a toll on your mental health" or "Sleep training makes it so much easier to cope." A narrative has emerged that babies are the source of a mother's mental health challenges and that children's needs should come second to the mother's mental health. This notion is often compared to the proverbial airplane oxygen mask that must go on us first before we can properly help anyone else.

While I agree that a mother's well-being is the source of a healthy family, and that society should be built around lifting her up in every way, I think that the definition of self-care for mental health has been

322

somewhat misconstrued. This is partially due to trending topics on social media and is a result of predatory marketing that is constantly trying to sell us a quick-fix solution to any challenge we may face.

What if the "oxygen mask" we as mothers need to put on first is not the sleep training, the formula, or the screen time, but rather the commitment to our inner healing so we can expand our capacity to meet our children's deepest needs without it breaking us? Mental fortitude is not achieved through lack of hardship but in our ability to face it and grow from it so we can be strong enough to allow our children's needs to come first. Every challenge we face is there as an opportunity to propel our growth.

The Mama Redirect

This week I offer you two simple tools for shifting your mindset. The first is simply through being mindful of the language you use and the stories you tell. Notice the difference you feel when you say, "My child is giving me a hard time" versus "My child is having a hard time." One makes you the victim while the other brings you to a place of compassion. Next time you're in the thick of it, try shifting from "I am miserable and exhausted right now and can't seem to do anything right" to "Today is inviting me to grow more resilient and patient. It's uncomfortable and challenging, but I know it's part of the process and I am capable of navigating it."

The second tool uses the term *redirect*, which is used to describe the parenting technique of helping your child redirect from a meltdown. By guiding their attention elsewhere, you can help them regulate big emotions. This is a method you will become very familiar with as a parent over the years, but I want you to become just as good at redirecting yourself, because sometimes it's us parents who need a redirect more than our children. My go-to redirects are living room dance parties, a warm bath, a massage, being with friends, eye gazing with my baby, fresh air, and sunshine. Make a list of your top Mama Redirects and use them to help you shake it off.

CONSCIOUS PARENTING

WITH JESSICA SILVER

This week I asked one of my best friends, Jessica Silver, to walk us through an inner child exploration. Jessica is a specialist in somatic therapy as well as a certified transformative bodywork practitioner with a master's degree in clinical psychology. Over the years, Jessica has held me through the most challenging seasons of my life and helped me move through immense grief and anger, which greatly prepared me for parenthood. When she became pregnant, I had the privilege of supporting her as her doula while I was twenty weeks pregnant myself.

Jessica's first year of motherhood was harder than most. Her daughter had a protein milk allergy and severe eczema and was hospitalized at four months. Her grace through it all and commitment to her daughter's health and healing were inspiring to witness and speak volumes to the work she does.

325

The concept of "inner child work" is a powerful therapeutic tool for personal growth, as it involves reconnecting and healing the wounded, vulnerable, and emotional aspects within us by revisiting and addressing our past experiences. As mothers learn to heal their own childhood wounds and learn to parent their children from a more empowered space, they will break cycles of intergenerational trauma for their family. Maintaining a healthy nervous system is a transformative gift that we can give to our children because our mood sets the emotional tone of our child's reality. Our children see us as energy and remember us as energy; as mothers, we need to take care of our nervous system.

When a mother feels grounded and confident that she can navigate the highs and lows of emotionality, she can encourage her children to feel their emotions freely and to listen to the wisdom that comes from them. She will feel equipped to face her child's big feelings with emotional stability. A regulated parent is a safe parent. When a child feels unsafe to experience the fullness of their feelings, they creatively and instinctually create defense mechanisms that allow them to turn away from the truth of how they feel to cope with their reality. I like to conceptualize "conscious parenting" as having a safe emotional connection with yourself, your child, and your inner child. When a child feels safe, they can bring the fullness of their spirit to the present moment rather than modulating their behavior to take care of their parent's feelings.

We all have an inner child or inner children within ourselves. These children are not literal children, but they represent the visceral and emotional

326

memories of the younger versions of ourselves throughout life. We refer to them as "children" because we can reflect on their vulnerabilities and lovingly re-mother them as the adults we are today. By revisiting the past and acknowledging the pain, neglect, or trauma that was experienced, we can release pent-up emotions and find closure. Unresolved childhood traumas and unmet needs often continue to subconsciously influence our behavior and emotions throughout adulthood. No matter our age, we all possess the emotions, thoughts, memories, and experiences from our life. Even if our minds may not be able to quickly recall, our bodies never forget what we have been through. As humans, we are brilliantly designed to survive and run our energy efficiently. If there is a part of us that feels unsafe, even from childhood, we will continue to invest energy into protecting that part of us until we truly feel that we are no longer under threat. Our inner children often hold these memories, and the only person who can truly heal them is the person who we are today.

For example, if a young girl grows up with an out-of-control parent who yelled and expressed their anger in ways that made everyone in the home feel unsafe, then she might have learned that the best way to protect herself was to run and hide. Fast-forward to the present day and that girl is now a mother to a toddler who is screaming and throwing tantrums. If she has never examined her childhood and coping skills from her past, then she may feel very confused as to why she is so uncomfortable with her toddler's intense expression of anger. During these times, she may feel triggered and have the strong urge to avoid, run away, and hide. Inner child work provides her the tools to differentiate between her own historical feelings of panic that are incongruent to the situation at hand and her actual feelings as a mother as she witnesses her child's meltdown.

Another example is if a young girl was raised by a parent who was depressed and sullen, then she might've learned that it is her job to make them happy and feel better again. Then, she grows up to be an adult who is stuck in unconscious people-pleasing behavior and doesn't know why she always takes

327

care of others before listening to her own needs. As a mother, when her baby is distressed and she can't immediately alleviate their suffering, she might feel old feelings of failure and unworthiness.

In both scenarios, we can see how the mother's brain gets hijacked into survival mode because her child's emotional intensity tugs on the trauma of her own past experiences. As much as she wants to be a safe place for her child, it may be difficult when she feels out of control herself. The magic of inner child work shows up when she learns to reconnect with her own wounded inner child and provide a reparative experience in real time so that she can regulate her nervous system. Within minutes, she can manage to bring her brain back online from a trauma state and into a place where she is able to feel safe enough to hold space for all parts of herself and her own child.

Mothering Your Inner Child

WITH JESSICA SILVER

Let's explore an exercise where you can identify how your own inner child shows up within your motherhood journey. Create safety in the context of this exercise by choosing an experience where you feel safe enough to navigate the memory on your own.

Close your eyes and remember a time in your parenting journey when you felt overwhelmed with challenging and intense emotions. This could be a single memory or a period of time. Call forward what happened, how you felt, and what was going on.

Pause here and take some breaths to give your body time to remember and remind yourself that you are safe and we are in an exercise of compassionate exploration. Now, focus on your physical sensations within your body and breathe into the parts that you feel are getting activated (e.g., areas that are contracting or growing in tension).

Then, ask yourself: "Is this the first time I've ever felt this way? Is this a familiar feeling from my past? Do I remember feeling this way when I was a child?" Write down whatever is coming up for you and which age(s) comes to mind.

Now, return to that memory and recall how you were treated when you felt that way. Were your feelings allowed to be? Did you have anyone safe you could turn toward to process? Did you have to hide your feelings to take care of someone else's feelings? Could you express them freely and spontaneously? Were you taught that it was a strength to push through or praised for not losing control? If it is difficult to remember, just focus on how this prompt made you feel. How comfortable were you to reexperience those feelings? What was your inner dialogue? Take some time to reflect and write down what came up for you.

Begin to imagine that you are connecting with your younger self as the parent you are today. Call her forward and see her exactly as she enters your visualization. Take time to really take her in; what is she wearing, how does she look at you, how does she truly feel? Try to see her through eyes of compassion. Feel that it is your sincere honor to be able to meet her from a place of acceptance, safety, and love. From that lens, lovingly put your hand over the areas where you feel tension building and begin to take deep, intentional breaths directly into the center of it.

Imagine that with each breath, you are leading the way and breathing together with your inner child. Now, you are co-regulating your nervous systems together. Your lungs are her lungs. Your heartbeat is her heartbeat. Show her that you welcome her to feel exactly how she feels and that you are so proud of her. Speak to your younger self from your heart and reflect back to her what you see (for example, "I see that you are afraid, angry, and overwhelmed"). Let her know that she is no longer alone. Say, "I am with you now and you are safe in my care. It's an honor to breathe with you, to hold you until these feelings pass, and there is no one in the world who knows how to comfort you more than me. I'm so sorry if you have felt alone for so long. I am here with you now and for the rest of our lives."

Once you initiate this connection with your inner child, it will always be established. You might need to check in with her multiple times a day or whenever you feel that old wounds are being triggered in your present-day reality. This is your opportunity to be the parent to yourself that you might have never had, to mother yourself from the inside out. It all begins with re-mothering your inner child to create a sense of safety in your own body and then being able to give that gift to the rest of the world.

A YEAR OF MOTHERING

Fourteen weeks postpartum coincides with the hundredth day of parenting your baby earthside! In Chinese culture, this milestone calls for a big celebration.[88] Baby is adorned in gold bracelets and showered with gifts to symbolize good luck. I find it really special that this hundredth day falls around the year anniversary of conception for most. One hundred days of mothering is a huge feat, but in reality, you have been mothering for a full year! Although your baby is only considered to be three and a half months old, today marks one year of growing your baby, holding your baby, and embodying the divine mother you are.

Your body has been instinctively nourishing and working hard every day for this past year to transform a poppy-sized embryo into a big-little human. Pregnancy is the chapter of parenthood when we're most connected to our innate nurturing wisdom that provides for our child without thought. Just as a tree knows how to grow leaves and the sun knows how to set, we know how to mother before we even know we've conceived. When a newborn crosses the threshold, your role as a mother evolves, but these powerful innate qualities remain. You are everything your baby needs and more just as you are.

Before you close the book, I want to leave you with one last nugget of wisdom to remember . . . That feeling that you have been changed forever on a cellular level, the feeling that you carry you child within your heart, is not just a sentiment. It has been scientifically validated through the study of Microchimerism. Mothers retain in their bodies the fetal cells from every pregnancy, forever. You have been transformed and the unbreakable bond with your baby is deeply engrained within your body for life.

ADDITIONAL RESOURCES

www.carson-meyer.com
www.carson-meyer.com/doula-resources
www.candthemoon.com

BOOKS

Anti-D Explained, by Sara Wickham

Birth as an American Rite of Passage,
by Robbie Davis-Floyd

The Book of Lymph,
by Lisa Levitt Gainsley

The First Forty Days, by Heng Ou

Having Faith, by Sandra Steingraber

The Mindful Mom-to-Be,
by Lori Bregman

Nourishing Traditions, by Sally Fallon

Placenta: The Forgotten Chakra,
by Robin Lim

Pushed, by Jennifer Block

Real Food for Pregnancy,
by Lily Nichols

Safe Infant Sleep, by James McKenna

The Tools, by Phil Stutz and Barry Michels

Transformed by Birth,
by Britta Bushnell

Your Baby, Your Way,
by Jennifer Margulis

WEBSITES

BelliBind

Breech Without Borders

Evidence Based Birth

EWG's Skin Deep Database

Go Diaper Free

Indie Birth

International Cesarean Awareness Network

Little Honey Money

Midwife Thinking

Physicians for Informed Consent

Sara Wickham

Weston Price Foundation

FILMS

American Circumcision

The Business of Being Born

The Milky Way

Why Not Home?

PODCASTS

Birth Instincts

Down to Birth

Informed Pregnancy

ACKNOWLEDGMENTS

I am in deep gratitude to every mother and child who has invited me to walk beside them as their doula. You are my greatest teachers, and getting to witness your strength and the divine moment of transformation is something I will never take for granted.

Thank you to Ricki Lake and Abby Epstein for making the film that rocked my world and ignited the spark within. To Hayley Oakes for planting the doula seed and to Lori Bregman for taking me under your wing and helping me grow to be the doula I am today. Lori, you model confidence, generosity, and true support of women like no other. I couldn't ask for a greater mentor. Thank you to Cristina Carlino for being a mentor and cheerleader in all my pursuits.

I am so very grateful to Carrie Battan, who flew out to Asheville to do a profile on homebirth for *Elle*. She approached my work and the topic with an open mind and integrity. Her article landed at Chronicle and is the reason this book came to be. Just weeks before giving birth to Lou, I found an email that had gone unnoticed in my spam box from Cara Bedick at Chronicle. I was convinced it was spam because it seemed too good to be true. Cara, Rachel, and the amazing team at Chronicle, thank you for making this dream a reality. Thank you for being the most magnificent book doulas.

Thank you to my agents at CAA, Cindy Uh and Abby Walters, for being there for me every step of the way.

Special thanks to Aleks Evanguilidi for walking with Lou, Johnathan, and me through pregnancy and passing on so much of your midwifery knowledge and rituals that has made me a healthier mama and a better doula.

I am forever grateful to Cait Turner for holding us through the birth portal with such profound grace and trust. I know that the universe led us to you for a reason. Your presence was a gift to our family.

Thank you, Annie Whitehouse, for finding us when we needed you most and taking such great care of our Lou.

Thanks to Noelle Kovary, Bella Baily, Aleiela Allen, Erica Mock, and Annie for sharing your recipes. You ladies know that food is my love sign.

I am deeply grateful to Jessica Silver-Thomas, Lisa Levitt Gainsley, Maura Moynihan, and Allison Oswald for contributing to this book and inspiring me in so many ways. Your wisdom has had such a profound impact on my life. Thank you for allowing me to share your gifts with others.

To my sisters Jennifer and Sarah and my brother Eli. I love you three so much and thank my lucky stars to be on this ride with you. Thank you for always being there to make everything better and for being my first line of support no matter what.

Thank you, Mom and Dad, for bringing me earthside to the greatest family and life and for surrounding me in love.

And to my favorite writer of all time, Johnathan Rice. Thank you for nourishing me (with love, humor, and food) 365 days of the year. Thank you for being the best father to our Lou and creating a magical life with us and for us. There is no way I could have written this book in the first year of parenthood without your dedication to our family.

Lou, thank you for choosing me as your mama, for expanding my heart more than I ever thought possible, and for giving me the greatest purpose in life.

To the nurses, midwives, OBs, and doulas supporting women in their power, I bow down to you!

337

ABOUT THE AUTHOR

Carson Meyer is a doula and certified nutrition consultant who has supported hundreds of women on their path to parenthood. She hosts circles for families across the country to help them access community and information on healthy pregnancy, birth, and post-partum practices. She also leads mentorship opportunities for new and aspiring doulas. Her work has been featured in *Elle*, *Vogue*, *GOOP*, and *Los Angeles Times*.

Carson is the founder of C & The Moon, a clean skin care line founded on the belief that the way we care for ourselves is intrinsically linked to the way we care for the planet.

She graduated from NYU's Gallatin School of Individualized Study in 2016 and lives in western North Carolina with her husband, Johnathan, their daughter, Lou, and Bernedoodle, Paulie.

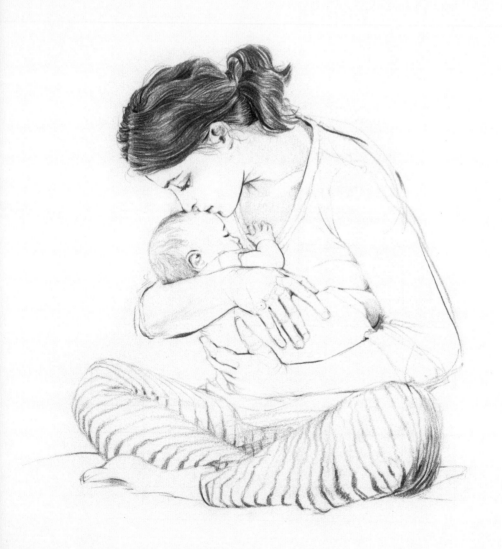

ENDNOTES

Introduction

1   Menard, K. M., S. L. Clark, J. P. Elliott, et al. "Cesarean Delivery Rates in the United States: The 1990s." *Obstetrics and Gynecology Clinics of North America* 26(2): 275–86, June 1, 1999. https://www.sciencedirect.com/science/article/abs /pii/S0889854505700747.

2   Tikkanen, R., M. Z. Gunja, M. FitzGerald, and L. C. Zephyrin. "Maternal Mortality and Maternity Care in the United States Compared to 10 Other Developed Countries." Commonwealth Fund, November 18, 2020. https://www.commonwealthfund.org/publications /issue-briefs/2020/nov/maternal-mortality-maternity -care-us-compared-10-countries.

3   Kenney, A M., A. Torres, N. Dittes, and J. Macias. "Medicaid Expenditures for Maternity and Newborn Care in America." *Family Planning Perspectives* 18(4): 196, July–August 1986. https://pubmed.ncbi.nlm.nih.gov/3100323.

4   Oi, M. "How Much Do Women around the World Pay to Give Birth?" BBC News, February 13, 2015. https://www .bbc.com/news/business-31052665.

5   Mohamoud, Y. A., E. Cassidy, E. Fuchs, et al. "Vital Signs: Maternity Care Experiences—United States, April 2023." Centers for Disease Control and Prevention, August 31, 2023. https://www.cdc.gov/mmwr/volumes/72/wr /mm7235e1.htm.

6   Flamm, B. L. "Cesarean Delivery in the United States: A Summary of the Past 20 Years." *Clinical Perspectives in Obstetrics and Gynecology.* New York: Springer, 1995. https://link.springer.com/chapter/10.1007/978-1-4612 -2482-2_1.

7   "Doctors Need More Nutrition Education." Harvard T. H. Chan School of Public Health News, 2017. https://www .hsph.harvard.edu/news/hsph-in-the-news/doctors -nutrition-education.

My Birth Story

8   Gao, L., E. Rabbitt, et al. "Steroid Receptor Coactivators 1 and 2 Mediate Fetal-to-Maternal Signaling That Initiates Parturition." *Journal of Clinical Investigation* 125(7): 2808–2824, July 1, 2015.

Week 4

9   Soma-Pillay, P., C. Nelson-Piercy, H. Tolppanen, and A. Mebazaa. "Physiological Changes in Pregnancy." *Cardiovascular Journal of Africa* 27(2): 89–94, March–April 2016. https://www.ncbi.nlm.nih.gov/pmc/articles/PMC4928162.

10   Mierzyński, R., E. Poniedziałek-Czajkowska, M. Sotowski, and M. Szydełko-Gorzkowicz. "Nutrition as Prevention Factor of Gestational Diabetes Mellitus: A Narrative Review." *Nutrients* 13(11): 3787, November 2021. https://www.ncbi.nlm.nih.gov/pmc/articles/PMC8625817.

11   Skolmowska, D., D. Głąbska, A. Kołota, and D. Guzek. "Effectiveness of Dietary Interventions to Treat Iron-Deficiency Anemia in Women: A Systematic Review of Randomized Controlled Trials." *Nutrients* 14(13): 2724, July 2022. https://www.ncbi.nlm.nih.gov/pmc/articles /PMC9268692.

12   Burchakov, D. I., I. V. Kuznetsova, and Y. B. Uspenskaya. "Omega-3 Long-Chain Polyunsaturated Fatty Acids and Preeclampsia: Trials Say 'No,' but Is It the Final Word?" *Nutrients* 9(12): 1364, December 2017. https://www.ncbi.nlm .nih.gov/pmc/articles/PMC5748814.

13   Marshall, N. E., B. Abrams, L. A. Barbour, et al. "The Importance of Nutrition in Pregnancy and Lactation: Lifelong Consequences." *American Journal of Obstetrics and Gynecology* 226(5): 607–32, May 2022. https://www.ncbi.nlm .nih.gov/pmc/articles/PMC9182711.

14   Dean, L. "Methylenetetrahydrofolate Reductase Deficiency." *Medical Genetics Summaries*, October 27, 2016. https://www.ncbi.nlm.nih.gov/books/NBK66131.

15   Scaglione, F., and G. Panzavolta. "Folate, Folic Acid and 5-Methyltetrahydrofolate Are Not the Same Thing." *Xenobiotica* 44(5): 480–88, May 2014. https://pubmed.ncbi.nlm .nih.gov/24494987.

16   Blusztajn, J. K., B. E. Slack, and T. J. Mellott. "Neuroprotective Actions of Dietary Choline." *Nutrients* 9(8): 815, August 2017. https://www.ncbi.nlm.nih.gov/pmc/articles /PMC5579609.

17   Carriquiry, A., and K. L. Schalinske. "Choline in the Diets of the U.S. Population: NHANES, 2003–2004." *The FASEB Journal* 21, January 2007. https://www.researchgate.net /publication/285738596_Choline_in_the_diets_of_the_ United_States_population_NHANES_2003-2004.

18   Zeisel, S. H., and K.-A. da Costa. "Choline: An Essential Nutrient for Public Health." *Nutrition Reviews* 67(11): 615–23, November 2009. https://www.ncbi.nlm.nih.gov /pmc/articles/PMC2782876.

19   "Vitamin A and Carotenoids." NIH Office of Dietary Supplements, 2023. https://ods.od.nih.gov/factsheets /VitaminA-HealthProfessional.

Week 5

20   Dekker, R. "The Evidence on: Due Dates." *Evidence Based Birth*, July 9, 2023. https://evidencebasedbirth.com/evidence -on-due-dates.

21   Margulies, M. "Should Pregnant Women Be Induced at 39 Weeks?" *Washington Post*, June 27, 2016. https://www .washingtonpost.com/national/health-science/should -pregnant-women-be-induced-at-39-weeks/2016/06/27 /e1bb9d16-27fe-11e6-b989-4e5479715b54_story.html.

22 Dekker, R. "Evidence on: Doulas." *Evidence Based Birth*, July 9, 2023. https://evidencebasedbirth.com/the-evidence-for-doulas.

23 Preis, H. A., B. B. Mahaffey, M. A. Lobel, and C. C. Heiselman. "The Impacts of the COVID-19 Pandemic on Birth Satisfaction in a Prospective Cohort of 2,341 U.S. Women." *Women and Birth* 35(5): 458–65, September 2022. https://www.sciencedirect.com/science/article/pii/S1871519221001761.

24 Zhou, J., K. L. Havens, C. P. Starnes, et al. "Changes in Social Support of Pregnant and Postnatal Mothers during the COVID-19 Pandemic." *Midwifery* 103, December 2021. https://www.ncbi.nlm.nih.gov/pmc/articles/PMC8485715.

25 "4 Common Pregnancy Complications." Johns Hopkins Medicine, November 1, 2022. https://www.hopkinsmedicine.org/health/conditions-and-diseases/staying-healthy-during-pregnancy/4-common-pregnancy-complications.

Week 7

26 Schwartz, J., and E. P. Simon. "Medical Hypnosis for Hyperemesis Gravidarum." *Birth* 26(4): 248–54, December 1999. https://pubmed.ncbi.nlm.nih.gov/10655831.

27 Glas, K. L. "Individualised Homeopathic Treatment of Nausea and Vomiting in the First Trimester and of COVID-19 in the Third Trimester of Pregnancy: A Case Report." *Homeopathy* 111(3): 202–209, August 2022. https://www.ncbi.nlm.nih.gov/pmc/articles/PMC9307322.

28 "Moderate Daily Caffeine Intake During Pregnancy May Lead to Smaller Birth Size." National Institutes of Health, March 25, 2021. https://www.nih.gov/news-events/news-releases/moderate-daily-caffeine-intake-during-pregnancy-may-lead-smaller-birth-size.

29 Ibid.

Week 9

30 Harley, K. G., K. L. Parra, B. Eskenazi, et al. "Reducing Phthalate, Paraben, and Phenol Exposure from Personal Care Products in Adolescent Girls: Findings from the Hermosa Intervention Study." *Environmental Health Perspectives* 124(10): 1600–7, October 2016. https://pubmed.ncbi.nlm.nih.gov/26947464.

31 Zhang, H. "BPA Replacement Linked to Increased Cardiovascular Disease." EHN, February 22, 2022. https://www.ehn.org/bpa-replacement-2656483035.html.

32 Alberta, L., S. M. Sweeney, and K. Wiss. "Diaper Dye Dermatitis." *Pediatrics* 116(3), September 2005. https://pubmed.ncbi.nlm.nih.gov/16140691.

33 Kazemi, Z., E. Aboutaleb, A. Shahsavani, et al. "Evaluation of Pollutants in Perfumes, Colognes and Health Effects on the Consumer: A Systematic Review." *Journal of Environmental Health Science & Engineering* 20(1): 589–98, June 2022. https://www.ncbi.nlm.nih.gov/pmc/articles/PMC9163252.

34 Tjalvin, G., et al. "Maternal Preconception Occupational Exposure to Cleaning Products and Disinfectants and Offspring Asthma." *Journal of Allergy and Clinical Immunology*, 149(1): 422–31, January 2022. https://www.sciencedirect.com/science/article/pii/S0091674921013993.

35 "EWG's 2024 Shopper's Guide to Pesticides in Produce." Environmental Working Group. https://www.ewg.org/foodnews/summary.php.

36 Richardson, B. A. "Sudden Infant Death Syndrome: A Possible Primary Cause." *Journal of the Forensic Science Society* 34(3): 199–204, July–September 1994. https://pubmed.ncbi.nlm.nih.gov/7523575.

Week 10

37 Cassidy, T. *Birth: The Surprising History of How We Are Born.* New York: Grove Press, 2007.

38 Rice, K. "Trends in Labor Induction in the United States, 1989 to 2020." *MCN: The American Journal of Maternal/Child Nursing* 47(4): 235, July/August 2022. https://journals.lww.com/mcnjournal/citation/2022/07000/trends_in_labor_induction_in_the_united_states,.13.aspx.

39 Petrullo, J. "United States Has Highest Infant, Maternal Mortality Rates despite the Most Health Care Spending." *AJMC*, January 31, 2023. https://www.ajmc.com/view/us-has-highest-infant-maternal-mortality-rates-despite-the-most-health-care-spending.

40 Beck, C. T., S. Watson, and R. K. Gable. "Traumatic Childbirth and Its Aftermath: Is There Anything Positive?" *Journal of Perinatal Education* 27(3), June 2018. https://www.ncbi.nlm.nih.gov/pmc/articles/PMC6193358.

Week 11

41 Newnham, J. P. "Effects of Frequent Ultrasound During Pregnancy: A Randomised Controlled Trial." *Lancet* 342(8876), October 9, 1993. https://pubmed.ncbi.nlm.nih.gov/8105165.

42 Ewigman, B. G. "Effect of Prenatal Ultrasound Screening on Perinatal Outcome. Radius Study Group." *New England Journal of Medicine* 329(12): 821–27, 1996. https://pubmed.ncbi.nlm.nih.gov/8355740.

43 Ibid.

44 Campbell, J D, et al. "Case-Control Study of Prenatal Ultrasonography Exposure in Children with Delayed Speech." *CMAJ : Canadian Medical Association Journal = Journal de l'Association Medicale Canadienne*, vol. 149, no. 10, 1993, pp. 1435–40, www.ncbi.nlm.nih.gov/pmc/articles/PMC1485930/. Accessed 29 Feb. 2024.

45 Kieler, H. "Sinistrality - a Side-Effect of Prenatal Sonography: A Comparative Study of Young Men." *Epidemiology* 12(6): 618–23, November 2001. https://pubmed.ncbi.nlm.nih.gov/11679787.

46 Sinatra, S. T., D. S. Sinatra, S. W. Sinatra, and G. Chevalier. "Grounding—The Universal Anti-Inflammatory Remedy." *Biomedical Journal* 46(1): 11–16, February 2023. https://www.ncbi.nlm.nih.gov/pmc/articles/PMC10105021.

Week 14

47 "Iron." Office of Dietary Supplements, National Institutes of Health, 2023. https://ods.od.nih.gov/factsheets/Iron -HealthProfessional.

48 Miko, E., A. Csaszar, J. Bodis, and K. Kovacs. "The Maternal-Fetal Gut Microbiota Axis: Physiological Changes, Dietary Influence, and Modulation Possibilities." *Life* 12(3): 424, March 2022. https://www.ncbi.nlm.nih.gov /pmc/articles/PMC8955030.

Week 17

49 Mercer, J. S., and R. L. Skovgaard. "Neonatal Transitional Physiology: A New Paradigm." *Journal of Perinatal & Neonatal Nursing* 15(4): 56–75, March 2002. https://pubmed .ncbi.nlm.nih.gov/11911621.

50 Andersson, O., B. Lindquist, and M. Lindgren. "Effect of Delayed Cord Clamping and Neurodevelopment at 4 Years of Age." *JAMA Pediatrics* 169(7): 631–38, July 2015. https://jamanetwork.com/journals/jamapediatrics /fullarticle/2296145.

51 Andersson, O., and J. S. Mercer. "Cord Management of the Term Newborn." *Clinics in Perinatology* 48(3): 447–70, August 2021. https://www.sciencedirect.com/science /article/pii/S0095510821000415.

52 Mercer, J. S., R.L. Skovgaard, J. Peareara-Eaves, and T. A. Bowman. "Nuchal Cord Management and Nurse-Midwifery Practice." *Journal of Midwifery & Women's Health* 50(5): 373–79, September–October 2005. https://pubmed .ncbi.nlm.nih.gov/16154063.

53 Masad, R., G. Gutvirtz, T. Wainstock, and E. Sheiner. "The Effect of Nuchal Cord on Perinatal Mortality and Long-Term Offspring Morbidity." *Nature News*, October 8, 2019. https://www.nature.com/articles/s41372-019-0511-x?fbclid =IwAR0Zpd2bJWEnuZm4gS5WPye8qAnl47w26JLarjS -oYk9DBuT9SxDeSmK_eU.

54 Zhang, Sarah. "Don't Pay for Cord-Blood Banking." *The Atlantic*, 17 Oct. 2022, www.theatlantic.com/health /archive/2022/10/cord-blood-banking-transplant-cost -worth-it/671765/.

55 Leung, P. C. "Placenta and Umbilical Cord in Traditional Chinese Medicine." *Regenerative Medicine Using Pregnancy-Specific Biological Substances*. New York: Springer, 2010. https://link.springer.com/chapter/10.1007/978-1-84882 -718-9_3.

56 Moyer, H. S. "The Power of Placenta." *Midwifery Today* 112, Winter 2015. https://www.midwiferytoday.com/mt-articles /the-power-of-placenta.

Week 20

57 Saftlas, A. F., L. Rubenstein, K. Prater, et al. "Cumulative Exposure to Paternal Seminal Fluid Prior to Conception and Subsequent Risk of Preeclampsia." *Journal of Reproductive Immunology* 101–102: 104–10, March 2014. https://pubmed.ncbi.nlm.nih.gov/24011785.

Week 21

58 Law, T. "Home Births Became More Popular During the Pandemic, but Many Insurers Still Don't Cover Them," *Time*, February 11, 2022. https://time.com/6145726/home -births-insurance-coverage.

Week 24

59 Dolatkhah, N., M. Hajifaraji, and S. K. Shakouri. "Nutrition Therapy in Managing Pregnant Women with Gestational Diabetes Mellitus: A Literature Review." *Journal of Family & Reproductive Health* 12(2): 57–72, June 2018. https://www.ncbi.nlm.nih.gov/pmc/articles/PMC6391302.

Week 26

60 Nilsson, U. "Soothing Music Can Increase Oxytocin Levels During Bed Rest After Open-Heart Surgery: A Randomised Control Trial." *Journal of Clinical Nursing* 18(15): 2153–61, August 2009.

Week 27

61 Dekker, R. "Friedman's Curve and Failure to Progress: A Leading Cause of Unplanned Cesareans." *Evidence Based Birth*, May 17, 2023. https://evidencebasedbirth.com /friedmans-curve-and-failure-to-progress-a-leading-cause -of-unplanned-c-sections.

62 Terreri, C. "What to Know about Your Water Breaking." Lamaze International, December 24, 2018. https://www .lamaze.org/Giving-Birth-with-Confidence/GBWC-Post /what-to-know-about-your-water-breaking.

63 Ibid.

Week 28

64 Heelan, L. "Fetal Monitoring: Creating a Culture of Safety with Informed Choice." *Journal of Perinatal Education* 22(3): 156–65, Summer 2013. https://www.ncbi.nlm.nih.gov/pmc /articles/PMC4010242/#jpe.1058-1243.22.3.bib06.024.

65 Boyle, A., U. M. Reddy, H. J. Landy, et al. "Primary Cesarean Delivery in the United States." *Obstetrics and Gynecology* 122(1): 33–40, July 2013. https://www.ncbi.nlm.nih.gov/pmc /articles/PMC3713634.

66 Coelho, G. D. P., L. F. A. Ayres, D. S. Barreto, et al. "Acquisition of Microbiota According to the Type of Birth: An Integrative Review." *Revista Latino-Americana de Enfermagem* 29, 2021. https://www.ncbi.nlm.nih.gov/pmc/articles /PMC8294792.

67 Mueller, N. T., E. Bakacs, J. Combellick, et al. "The Infant Microbiome Development: Mom Matters." *Trends in Molecular Medicine* 21(2): 109–17, February 2015. https://www.ncbi .nlm.nih.gov/pmc/articles/PMC4464665.

Week 29

68 "Safety Information for Hepatitis B Vaccines." Centers for Disease Control and Prevention, January 16, 2024. https:// www.cdc.gov/vaccinesafety/vaccines/hepatitis-b-vaccine .html#:~:text=The%20most%20common%20side%20effects ,heartbeat%2C%20dizziness%2C%20and%20weakness.

343

Week 30

69 Castro-Vasquez, B. A., and C. Taboada. "Accuracy of Estimated Fetal Weight in Third Trimester." *Obstetrics & Gynecology* 135: 16S–17S, May 2020. https://journals.lww .com/greenjournal/abstract/2020/05001/accuracy_of _estimated_fetal_weight_in_third.54.aspx.

70 Dekker, R. "What Is the Evidence for Induction or C-Section for a Big Baby?" *Evidence Based Birth*, June 5, 2013, https://evidencebasedbirth.com/evidence-for -induction-or-c-section-for-big-baby/.

Week 31

71 Dekker, R. "The Evidence on: Waterbirth." *Evidence Based Birth*, July 8, 2014. https://evidencebasedbirth.com /waterbirth.

72 Xu, C., X. Wang, X. Chi, et al. "Association of Epidural Analgesia during Labor and Early Postpartum Urinary Incontinence among Women Delivered Vaginally: A Propensity Score Matched Retrospective Cohort Study." *BMC Pregnancy and Childbirth* 23, September 16, 2023. https:// www.ncbi.nlm.nih.gov/pmc/articles/PMC10504782.

73 Dekker, R. "Effects of IV Opioids during Labor." *Evidence Based Birth*, March 20, 2018. https://evidencebasedbirth .com/effects-of-iv-opioids-during-labor.

Week 32

74 "Sudden and Unexpected Deaths in Infancy and Childhood." National Child Mortality Database, December 8, 2022. https://www.ncmd.info/publications/sudden -unexpected-death-infant-child.

Week 33

75 "Is It Normal to Have a Veiny Penis?" *Medical News Today*, August 14, 2019. https://www.medicalnewstoday.com /articles/326037#summary.

76 Marshall, R. E., W. C. Stratton, J. A. Moore, and S. B. Boxerman. "Circumcision I: Effects Upon Newborn Behavior." *Infant Behavior and Development* 3: 1–14, January 1980. https://doi.org/10.1016/S0163-6383(80)80003-8.

Week 34

77 Sarris, Jerome, et al. "Nutritional Medicine as Mainstream in Psychiatry." *The Lancet Psychiatry*, vol. 2, no. 3, Mar. 2015, pp. 271–274, www.thelancet.com/journals/lanpsy/article /PIIS2215-0366(14)00051-0/fulltext, https://doi.org/10.1016 /s2215-0366(14)00051-0. Accessed 4 Oct. 2019.

Week 36

78 Dekker, R. "The Evidence on: Group B Strep." *Evidence Based Birth*, July 26, 2023. https://evidencebasedbirth.com /groupbstrep.

Week 1 Earthside

79 Huang, J., Q. Zhao, J. Li, et al. "Correlation Between Neonatal Hyperbilirubinemia and Vitamin D Levels: A Meta-Analysis." *PLoS One* 16(5), May 27, 2021. https:// www.ncbi.nlm.nih.gov/pmc/articles/PMC8158937.

Week 3 Earthside

80 Hahn-Holbrook, J., and M. Haselton. "Is Postpartum Depression a Disease of Modern Civilization?" *Current Directions in Psychological Science* 23(6): 395–400, December 2014. https://www.ncbi.nlm.nih.gov/pmc/articles /PMC5426853.

81 Ibid.

82 Ghaedrahmati, M., A. Kazemi, G. Kheirabadi, et al. "Postpartum Depression Risk Factors: A Narrative Review." *Journal of Education and Health Promotion* 6, August 9, 2017. https://www.ncbi.nlm.nih.gov/pmc/articles/PMC5561681.

83 Etebary, S., S. Nikseresht, H. R. Sadeghipour, and M. R. Zarrindast. "Postpartum Depression and Role of Serum Trace Elements." *Iranian Journal of Psychiatry* 5(2): 40–46, 2010. https://pubmed.ncbi.nlm.nih.gov/22952489.

84 Ghaedrahmati, M., A. Kazemi, G. Kheirabadi, et al. "Postpartum Depression Risk Factors: A Narrative Review." *Journal of Education and Health Promotion* 6, August 9, 2017. https://www.ncbi.nlm.nih.gov/pmc/articles/PMC5561681.

Week 9 Earthside

85 Nichols, L. "The Truth about Postpartum Hair Loss." Lily Nichols RDN, September 28, 2023. https://lilynicholsrdn .com/truth-postpartum-hair-loss.

Week 11 Earthside

86 Care.com Editorial Staff. "This Is How Much Child Care Costs in 2021." *Care.com Resources*, 10 June 2021, www.care .com/c/how-much-does-child-care-cost/.

Week 12 Earthside

87 Stutz, Phil, and Barry Michels. *The Tools*. Random House, 29 May 2012.

Week 14 Earthside

88 "The Joyful Tradition of Gifting on 100 Days: Celebrating Milestones in Chinese Culture." *Lovingly Signed*, August 29, 2023. https://lovinglysigned.com.sg/blogs/news/the-joyful -tradition-of-gifting-on-100-days-celebrating-milestones -in-chinese-culture.